Community Health Nursing: A Practical Guide

Patricia L. Carroll RN, BC, CEN, RRT, MS
Educational Medical Consultants
Meriden, CT

Health Care Coordinator
Shelter Now
Meriden, CT

THOMSON

DELMAR LEARNING   Australia · Canada · Mexico · Singapore · Spain · United Kingdom · United States

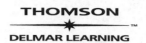

THOMSON

DELMAR LEARNING

Community Health Nursing: A Practical Guide
Patricia L. Carroll

Vice President Health Care Business Unit:
William Brottmiller

Editorial Director:
Cathy L. Esperti

Acquisitions Editor
Matthew Filimonov

Editorial Assistant:
Patricia Osborn

Production Editor:
James Zayicek

Executive Marketing Director:
Jennifer McAvey

For permission to use material from this text or product, contact us by
Tel (800) 730–2214
Fax (800) 720–2215
www.thomsonrights.com

Library of Congress Cataloging-in-Publication Data

Carroll, Patricia L.
  Community health nursing : a practical guide
/ Patricia L. Carroll.
    p. ; cm.
  Includes index.
  ISBN 0-7668-4139-1
  1. Community health nursing. I. Title.
  [DNLM: 1. Community Halth Nursing. WY 106 C319c 2004]
  RT98.C375 2004
  610.73'43—dc 21
                                        2003044003

Notice to the Reader

Publisher does not warrant or guarantee any of the products described herein or perform any independent analysis in connection with any of the production information contained herein. Publisher does not assume, and expressly disclaims, any obligation to obtain and include information other than that provided to it by the manufacturer.

The reader is expressly warned to consider and adopt all safety precautions that might be indicated by the activities described herein and to avoid all potential hazards. By following the instructions contained herein, the reader willingly assumes all risks in connection with such instructions.

The publisher makes no representations or warranties of any kind, including but not limited to, the warranties of fitness for particular purpose or merchantability, nor are any such representations implied with respect to the material set forth herein, and the publisher takes no responsibility with respect to such material. The publisher shall not be liable for any special, consequential, or exemplary damages resulting, in whole or part, from the reader's use of, or reliance upon, this material.

This book is dedicated to all the people who comprise the underserved populations that rely on the knowledge, compassion, and dedication of community health nurses every day.

CONTENTS

FOREWORD

I have practiced nursing for almost 30 years. As a diploma graduate, I did not have any formal community health content or clinical experience as a student since care was always provided in an institutional setting. During the first 10 years of my career I practiced in hospitals, outpatient clinics, and homes. Even though the settings were different, I had to learn (rather helter-skelter) the community health principles that had been neglected in my basic education. I decided that practicing in the community was my love. After completing my BSN, where I had a formal community health course and clinical experience, I went to the University of North Carolina School of Public Health for my master's degree in public health nursing and education.

I have spent the past two decades of my career teaching community health in several BSN programs and as an administrator, clinician, discharge planner, author, and now editor in home care. Throughout all of these experiences I have had the privilege of working with thousands of nurses. I continue to see how these practitioners must understand and use community health principles more than ever, regardless of what setting they practice in.

There has never been a time when community health nursing principles are more needed yet less understood by both practicing nurses and nursing students. As the U.S. population ages, there will be more demand for nurses to work directly in the community. Nurses choosing to practice in institutions will also need to be aware of how home, community, family, environment, and resources can be used to plan discharge efficiently and effectively.

Additionally, financial pressures of providing adequate care for all Americans will continue to be problematic. To meet long-term goals of cost savings while delivering the best care, new care methods must be created and likely will use community health principles to develop specialty programs and approaches to care for specific population groups.

The nursing profession is realizing the need to educate practitioners about these principles by including content on the NCLEX exams and integrating more community health content in associate degree and external degree programs. Many practicing nurses who did not have this content in their formal preparation are now being asked to apply these concepts to their current work situation, perhaps in the hospital, nursing home, or home. This has created a strong demand for a concise, comprehensive reference that can quickly address these educational needs.

I am proud to say that Pat Carroll has done an outstanding job of accomplishing what many would see as impossible—presenting the complex subject of community health nursing in a concise, outline format founded on principles that allows the reader to apply material to practice.

This book is an interactive experience that involves the reader immediately. Each chapter is presented in outline format with clear definitions and essential content divided under the major missions of community health nursing. References and a list of Web sites at the end of each chapter provide further information so knowledge is enhanced and the nurse can pursue further independent learning and consider how this material applies to practice.

A major strength of the book is the three types of questions presented in each chapter, which give the book flexibility to be used in the various ways the author has envisioned. The NCLEX-type review questions are multiple-choice with a single correct answer. The critical thinking questions relate to specific chapter content and help the reader apply content to situations in a short-answer format. These two sets of questions have answers provided at the back of the book to enhance learning. A challenging third set of community-specific discussion questions allows the content to be applied to local situations in the reader's own community.

Community health is a broad field requiring nurses to think holistically and environmentally yet focus on prevention and treatment. To form this holistic practice, the nurse must appreciate how the individual, family, community, nation, and the world affect health and illness. Since the events of September 11, 2001, it is clear nurses must be more involved in caring for all diseases that affect populations as well as planning and carrying out prevention of internal and external threats to our nation's well-being.

I believe that Pat Carroll's book is an important addition to the community health literature and that it will foster a higher standard of community health nursing practice as we find ways to keep the public's health our utmost concern and nurses constantly in the picture.

Carolyn J. Humphrey, RN, MS, MPH, FAAN
Editor, *Home Healthcare Nurse*
Louisville, KY

PREFACE

Community health nursing is both the rich heritage and the limitless future of contemporary nursing practice. The U.S. Public Health Service was created in 1902 and began a tradition of a health care system that recognizes health needs of special population groups. Missions of community health nursing include:

- health promotion
- health protection
- health balance
- disease prevention
- social justice

In the past 20 years, there has been a significant shift from institution-based care to community-based care for all population groups. At the same time, there have been ever-shifting priorities among population groups, including controlling infectious diseases such as HIV/AIDS, sexually transmitted diseases, SARS (severe acute respiratory syndrome), and multidrug-resistant tuberculosis; properly treating a variety of chronic mental illnesses, including substance abuse; providing services to the homeless and striving to help them find permanent homes; and working with families to encourage healthy interactions, enhance child development, and reduce domestic violence. In the fall of 2001, the nation's priorities shifted once more as we focused for the first time on terrorism and its health consequences on U.S. soil. In this book, you will learn about all of these topics and more. I have even devoted a special section about responding to terrorism (biological, chemical, nuclear, and incendiary weapons) so you can have a reliable reference on this critically important issue.

This book is designed to be used two ways: as a text for traditional nursing programs that prefer using a handbook of community health nursing rather than a full textbook; alternatively, as a comprehensive overview of this aspect of nursing practice for nurses in nontraditional nursing degree programs and those reviewing for class and the NCLEX exam.

Each chapter follows the same format to enhance learning:

- key terms for you to know (highlighted in the text)
- content in outline form, focusing on practical, need-to-know information
- multiple-choice review questions in NCLEX format
- critical-thinking questions that encourage you to apply key concepts you learned as you read the section
- community-specific discussion questions that you can use to apply concepts to your own community; these questions can form the basis of classroom assignments or study group work
- print reference list
- Web sources to encourage you to explore the latest trends and issues online
- answers to multiple-choice and critical-thinking questions so you can check your work

I am proud to be a registered nurse and I am delighted to have this opportunity to help you learn about community health nursing, which has become a special interest of mine. We cannot predict what the future holds, but I can assure you that community health nurses will continue to play a critical role in promoting, protecting, maintaining, and enhancing our nation's health and well-being far into the twenty-first century.

I would like to hear from you and learn what you liked best about this book, what you would like to see added, or what you might have had trouble with. You can visit my Web site at www.nursesnotebook.com or e-mail me at CH@nursesnotebook.com.

Here's to your success!

Patricia L. Carroll, RN,BC, CEN, RRT, MS
Meriden, CT

ACKNOWLEDGMENTS

While an author's name appears on the cover of a book, any author will tell you that getting a book into reader's hands is a team effort. Greatest appreciation to Matthew Filimonov, whose vision brought this book to life. He planted the seed and helped it grow into this reference you hold in your hands. I am delighted to thank my writing colleague and dear friend, Beth Richards, for her assistance in researching Web sites and for editing the manuscript. This is a better book because she was a part of the team. And a special nod to Carol Bifulco and her team at Bookcomp, Inc. Her patience with me showed no bounds, and for that I am grateful.

I would not be able to complete any project without the love and support of my husband, Bob. He understands why I sit at my computer writing when I would rather be on the couch with him. He is incredibly patient, considering all the time I spend writing and teaching and working to improve the care clients receive, whether it is in the hospital or in the community.

ABOUT THE AUTHOR

Patricia Carroll has more than 20 years' experience in health care as both a registered respiratory therapist and a registered nurse. She has worked in neonatal, pediatric, and adult critical care, medical-surgical, and high-tech home care, and has spent the past 12 years in clinical practice in emergency nursing. She spent most of 2002 laying the groundwork to be the volunteer coordinator of a wellness center at the homeless shelter that serves her community, and putting the principles discussed in this book into action.

She welcomes comments from faculty and students using this book. You can e-mail her from her Web site www.nursesnotebook.com.

REVIEWER LIST

Patty Leary, Med
Mecosta Osceola Career Center
Big Rapids, MI

Carol Vogt, DrPH, RN
Director of Health Service Management Program
Nursing Faculty Member
Cabarrus College of Health Sciences
Concord, NC

Janet Courtney, RN, MSN
Department of Nursing
Professor of Nursing
Holyoke Community College
Holyoke, MA

Linda Wood, RN, MSN
Director of Practical Nursing
Massanutten Technical Center
Harrisonburg, VA

Part I

What Is Community Health Nursing?

COMMUNITY HEALTH NURSING

community

community health nursing

disease prevention

downstream thinking

empowerment

health balance

health promotion

health protection

participation

population(s)

relationships

risk

social justice

upstream thinking

INTRODUCTION

Increasingly, nurses are being called upon to deliver care to individuals, families, and communities in a variety of settings and environments. This chapter introduces the many ways nurses are being called upon to practice outside of a traditional hospital or clinic setting by exploring the role, focus, and missions of a community health nurse.

KEY POINTS

1. **Community health nursing** preserves and improves the health of populations and communities worldwide by meeting the collective needs of the community and society.

   A.   A **population** is a statistical aggregate or subgroup of people with similar or identical characteristics.

   B.   A **community** is a group of people sharing common interests, needs, resources, and environments.

   C.   Populations and communities can be formed based on ethnic, economic, familial, geographic, religious, social, or other characteristics.

2. Community health nursing meets its goals by identifying problems (for example, a high incidence of hypertension in a particular population) and supporting community **participation** in the process of preserving and improving health.

   A.   Key characteristics of community health nursing

       i.   caring **relationships** and partnerships with families and communities. People in the community are seen as essential participants in the process of promoting health and preventing illness.

      ii.   The community health nurse as a participant and facilitator, rather than just a dispenser of medications or information. This approach differs from the one sometimes seen in the traditional health care environment.

     iii.   focus on empowerment of families and communities. **Empowerment** means finding ways for people in a community or population to acquire skills and knowledge so that they can participate in decision making about their health.

     iv.   mutual respect and cooperation from both the giver and the receiver of care. The implications of empowerment in a population are that empowered people and communities can:

         a. use their power effectively, acting as advocates for themselves

         b. create a system that works better for them than systems already in place

         c. develop new, creative resources and increase their own resourcefulness

         d. collaborate and cooperate within the community as well as with those outside the community

         e. work effectively with and respect diversity and differences

      v.   focus on populations or subpopulations rather than individual-based practice.

     vi.   **upstream thinking.** This type of thinking focuses on identifying and, if possible, changing the economic, political, social, and environmental variables that can contribute to poor health of a population or worldwide. Upstream thinking differs significantly from downstream thinking, the focus of much of the health care environment in the United States and many developed countries.

     vii. **downstream thinking.** This type of thinking focuses on individual interventions over the short term.

    viii. orientation toward identification of populations at risk. **Risk** is the probability that an event, outcome, disease, or condition will develop within a certain time frame.

B.   Missions of community health nursing

       i. **health promotion.** The World Health Organization (WHO) defines health promotion as actions related to lifestyles and choices that maintain or enhance a population's health.

         a. Health has multidimensional aspects, including physical health, mental health, and social and environmental health.

         b. Health promotion includes individuals' and communities' abilities to cope with changes (environmental, social) and to maintain overall health and well-being.

     ii. **health protection.** This includes activities designed to detect or prevent illness, or alter disease processes.

         a. Health protection also includes workplace safety and health, food and drug safety, and other health/safety areas, as well as regulations that provide for them.

         b. A major factor that distinguishes health protection from health promotion is that in health protection, individuals want to avoid illness and its consequences.

    iii. **health balance.** This is a state of well-being that results from a healthy interaction between a person's body, mind, spirit, and environment.

    iv. **disease prevention.** This includes activities designed to protect people from disease and its consequences. In community health nursing, there are three levels of disease prevention:

         a. primary (prevent a problem before it occurs)

         b. secondary (diagnose and treat a condition in its earliest stages, before it has a chance to become full-blown; this includes disease screening)

         c. tertiary (prevent further progression of a disease that has already occurred)

         d. These three levels of disease prevention will be discussed throughout this text, as they are essential components of all community health nursing activities.

     v. **social justice.** This concept states that all people have a right to certain "basics" of life, such as adequate income and health protection.

         a. When a population is not able to acquire these basic needs, other parts of the community (private, government, or a combination of both) may take collective action to make sure that these needs are met.

  b. This has traditionally been a key role of public or community health.

  vi. disease prevention and health promotion are not synonymous. They function on a continuum that stretches from health all the way to illness and disability.

C. Community health nurses contribute in the following ways to the missions of community health:

  i. help *develop a system of comprehensive health care* based on population-focused health promotion, health balance, health protection, disease prevention, and social justice—rather than individually focused disease prevention or control.

  ii. help *coordinate health care services,* recognizing that working with populations requires sharing of resources and coordination, and that populations at risk often do not have access to integrated care.

  iii. *provide health education services,* especially to vulnerable populations.

  a. A key focus of community health nursing is the prevention of disease before it causes illness and disability.

  b. Vulnerable populations often receive fewer preventive and educational services, and are more likely to be seen by the traditional individual-based health system only after a disease or illness has progressed.

  iv. *work in a variety of settings,* at a variety of levels.

  a. Settings can include schools, health care planning agencies in the community, neighborhood or community clinics, or senior centers. Some community health nurses also provide home-based care to at-risk populations such as pregnant teens.

  b. Levels of involvement can be person-to-person, person-to-group, as members of health care planning boards or councils, or in educational institutions.

  c. Community health nurses can also serve as elected officials or at commissioner or other levels in order to implement and impact community health policy.

REVIEW ACTIVITIES

Questions

1. For which types of clients is the community health nurse primarily responsible?

  a. individuals

  b. families

   c. populations

   d. geopolitical entities

2. As community health nurses engage in the process of community empowerment, it is essential that they:

   a. gather data for the community

   b. form partnerships with people in the community

   c. make decisions for people in the community

   d. accept responsibility for people's actions

3. A person with no known illness whose daily routine consists of walking and following a healthy diet would best be characterized as engaging in which kind of activities?

   a. health balance

   b. disease prevention

   c. health promotion

   d. self-fulfillment

4. A community health action that focuses on reducing frequency and severity of asthma attacks in inner-city children by requiring a local incinerator to install particulate filters is an example of:

   a. downstream thinking

   b. risk management

   c. primary prevention

   d. upstream thinking

5. A community that uses the resources of a neighborhood church to provide a latchkey children's program, to sponsor prayer/support groups for people who are ill, and to grow a community garden that sends vegetables to elderly shut-ins are engaged in what kind of activity?

   a. disease prevention

   b. health protection

   c. risk management

   d. health balance

6. A nursing activity designed to diagnose and treat a disease or condition in its earliest stages, before it becomes full-blown, would be classified as:

   a. primary prevention

   b. secondary prevention

   c. tertiary prevention

   d. health education

7. Which of the following is a contribution of community health nurses to the community's health?

   a. providing health education to vulnerable populations

   b. coordinating access to integrated care for a population

    c.   developing comprehensive systems of health care in a variety of settings

    d.   all of the above

8. In which of the following settings would a community health nurse be less likely to be involved?

    a.   neighborhood or community clinic or senior center

    b.   physician's office with focus on individual client care

    c.   home-based care

    d.   neighborhood planning board

Critical-Thinking Questions

1. Empowerment is a key concept for community health nursing. Discuss empowerment and describe its characteristics and implications. Provide an example of an empowered community or communities. What are the possible limitations of this concept?

2. For a community health problem such as HIV or drug-resistant tuberculosis, identify upstream thinking-based solutions and downstream thinking-based solutions that could be applied to the problems. What are the advantages and disadvantages of each type of thinking?

Discussion Questions

1. Describe in your own words the most significant issue that will influence community health nursing in your community in the twenty-first century.

2. What are the various community health care providers in your city or region? How do you know about them? What do they do?

3. Identify an at-risk population in your community. What are its key characteristics? What health events or diseases are likely in this population?

References

American Nurses Association. (1986). *Standards of community health nursing practice.* Washington, DC: American Nurses Association.

Doran, T. (2001). Policy and practice: Providing seamless community health and social services. *Br J Community Nurs, 6*(8), 387, 390–393.

Drevdahl, D., Dorcy, K. S., & Grevstad, L. (2001). Integrating principles of community-centered practice in a community health nursing practicum. *Nurse Educ, 26*(5), 234–239.

Hitchcock, J., Schubert, P., & Thomas, S. (1999). *Community health nursing: Caring in action.* Clifton Park, NY: Delmar Learning.

Johnson, M. O. (2001). Meeting health care needs of a vulnerable population: Perceived barriers. *J Community Health Nurs, 18*(1), 35–52.

Koch, T. & Kralik, D. (2001). Chronic illness: Reflections on a community-based action research programme. *J Adv Nurs., 40*(7), 330–333.

Web Sites

American Association for the History of Nursing
      http://www.aahn.org
American Journal of Public Health
      http://www.ajph.org/
American Nurses Association
      http://www.nursingworld.org
American Public Health Association
      http://www.apha.org/
Association of Asian Pacific Community Health Organizations (AAPCHO)
      http://www.aapcho.org/

Centers for Disease Control and Prevention
    http://www.cdc.gov (search for "community health")

Community Health Status Report, U.S. Department of Health and Human Services
    http://www.communityhealth.hrsa.gov/

Journal of Epidemiology and Community Health
    http://jech.bmjjournals.com/

World Health Organization (WHO)
    http://www.who.int

WWW Virtual Library on Public Health
    http://www.ldb.org.vl/

POPULATION-FOCUSED CARE

assessment

assets assessment

assurance

environmental hazards

epidemiological research

evaluation

health promotion

needs assessment

policy development

population-based approach

program planning

public health

risk

INTRODUCTION

Community health nurses are focused on populations rather than individuals. Nurses working with populations are broadly concerned with health promotion and the needs of a population or community rather than a specific individual. This chapter examines the components and factors that shape a community health nurse's perspective.

KEY POINTS

1. **Health promotion,** a key focus of community health nursing, enables people and communities to improve their health by increasing control over the

factors that contribute to health, as well as decreasing the impact of factors that contribute to absence of health. This includes enabling and empowering people to:

A.   recognize their own health needs
B.   develop their knowledge and skills and thus increase control over the actions that can impact their own health
C.   participate meaningfully in developing strategies to improve their own health care

2. A **population-based approach** requires a shift from the traditional focus on individual health needs to the needs of a community or population group or subgroup.

A.   This approach also emphasizes strategies for promoting and maintaining health, and preventing disease, with attention to the economic, social, and political environments of the community as they impact a community's health.
B.   Components of a population approach include:

  i.   **epidemiological research.** Epidemiology is the study of the distribution of illnesses or other health states in a population; sound research requires reliable data about a population.
  ii. **needs assessment.** This assessment includes systematically taking stock of what a community requires to maintain the best health for, or prevent or treat disease in, its members. All— providers, clients, and other key parties—must be included in the assessment.
  iii. **program planning.** This includes identifying the current situation or incident that needs improvement or change, indicating the desired outcome, and then designing a series of steps to move from the current situation to the desired situation.
  iv. **evaluation.** A systematic inquiry to determine if the program followed its plan and met its goals. Evaluation can cover the appropriateness of the program itself, or can assess the effectiveness of the process of carrying out the program goals.

C.   Health professionals and social scientists agree that many risk factors may be out of the control of individuals. **Risk** needs to be seen as part of the larger picture—local, national, and global systems (both natural and human-made).
D.   Community health practice and public health practice are closely related. Public health practice in the past 200 years has significantly improved the health status and life expectancy of the U.S. population. Some of these measures include:

     i. protecting the public from **environmental hazards.** These include:
- a. improving the quality of air and reducing pollution, especially in cities
- b. developing systems and protocols to process hazardous materials safely, keep drinking water supplies safe, and dispose of sewage safely and effectively
- c. developing measures and regulations to prevent work-related hazards and injuries

    ii. health promotion. This includes measures to help populations prevent the occurrence of disease, or to prevent disease from progressing. Examples are educating people about:
- a. the hazards of tobacco use and alcohol abuse
- b. how to control hypertension
- c. the links between lifestyle factors and chronic diseases such as heart disease or diabetes
- d. injury prevention, through safe use of tools, automobiles, bicycles, and so on

E. The core functions of public health are:

    i. **assessment:** The controlled, systematic collection of data, monitoring health conditions or events, and distributing information.

    ii. **policy development:** Using reliable, scientific assessment data to make public health decisions or set policy. Policy development also requires knowledge of a population and of how policy impacts health, and leadership skills to implement policy in a community.

    iii. **assurance:** Making sure that services are available to those who are not able to afford them through channels such as private health care providers.

F. **Public health** is essential in influencing population health and providing a foundation for health care systems.

G. In addition to planning service across the three levels of health care—primary, secondary, and tertiary—population-focused health care also plans based on needs assessment and assets assessment.

    i. needs assessment: systematic appraisal of the type, intensity, and nature of health needs as perceived by those in a given community

    ii. **assets assessment:** seeing populations in terms of the resources that they possess and acknowledging and using these assets

H. Public health has a historical focus on

    i. assessing and identifying subpopulations at high risk or threat of disease or at high risk of poor recovery

    ii. making sure resources and services are available and accessible to this population

REVIEW ACTIVITIES

Questions

1. A key component of health promotion is that people in a community are able to:
   a. access private health insurance to cover their medical expenses
   b. recognize their health needs and help develop strategies to improve their own health care
   c. stop activities such as smoking or alcohol consumption that are harmful to health
   d. none of the above

2. Which of the following is *not* a part of a population-based approach to community health care?
   a. focus on health needs of the whole community rather than just individuals
   b. attention to the economic, social, and political environments of the community
   c. needs assessment and planning
   d. minimizing preventive health care strategies

3. Effective epidemiological research requires:
   a. needs assessment, program planning, and evaluation
   b. statistical evidence drawn from expert sources outside the community
   c. a federal grant for funding the necessary paperwork and reports
   d. that the desired outcome not be identified until the study is complete, to avoid tainting the data

4. Epidemiological research is designed to:
   a. identify which parts of the population have poor hygiene
   b. study how illnesses or other health events are distributed throughout a population
   c. target minority ethnic groups
   d. find out which communities use their health care dollars wisely

5. Program planning is essential to community health efforts because it
   a. ensures continued government funding
   b. allows systematic identification of needs and outcomes, and development of action steps
   c. must happen before needs assessment
   d. keeps different constituent groups from disagreeing about activities or outcomes

6. Public health measures to protect the community/public from environmental hazards include:
   a. reducing air pollution in cities
   b. processing hazardous waste and sewage safely and effectively and keeping drinking water supplies safe
   c. reducing work-related injuries
   d. all of the above

7. What are the core functions of public health?
   a. assessment, policy development, and assurance
   b. assessment, policy development, and budgetary control
   c. development of national policies to decrease environmental toxins
   d. needs assessment, assets assessment, and assurance

Critical-Thinking Questions

1. Name three ways that a population could develop knowledge and skills that could in turn increase control over their own health. What strategies could this population develop to improve their own health care?

2. An epidemiological study is to be done concerning exposure-related illness (frostbite, foot infections) in the homeless population. Discuss how data could be gathered. What needs does this community have? How could such a program be evaluated?

3. How is policy development related to community health?

4. You have been asked to do an assets assessment for a group of recently arrived immigrants. What resources could you expect them to possess? How does your assets assessment differ from a needs assessment?

Discussion Questions

1. What are some of the health promotion strategies currently being used in your community?

2. Have any epidemiological studies been performed in your community? If so, what kind? What kind of agencies usually perform these studies? Where could you access this information?

3. What are the public health practices in place in your community designed to protect the public from environmental hazards such as pollution, hazardous materials, sewage, and work injuries? Do you know how effective these practices are? Has there been coverage recently in the local press concerning one or more of these hazards?

4. How aware are you of the educational health promotion activities in your community? How do people in your community learn about alcohol abuse? Smoking cessation workshops? Hypertension? Sexually transmitted diseases? Name some of the educational activities or presentations you have seen in the past six months.

References

American Nurses Association. (1986). *Standards of community health nursing practice.* Washington, DC: American Nurses Association.

Baldwin, K. A., Humbles, P. L., Armmer, F. A., & Cramer, M. (2001, September–October). Perceived health needs of urban African American church congregants. *Public Health Nurs, 18*(5), 295–303.

Bice-Stephens, W. (2001). Practical tips: Designing a learning-needs survey—10 steps to success. *J Contin Educ Nurs, 32*(4), 150–151.

Campbell, S. (2001). Assessing community healthcare needs: Lessons from Africa. *Nurs Stand, 15*(47), 41–44.

Hitchcock, J., Schubert, P., & Thomas, S. (1999). *Community health nursing: Caring in action.* Clifton Park, NY: Delmar Learning.

Web Sites

American Journal of Public Health
http://www.ajph.org/

American Nurses Association
http://www.nursingworld.org

American Public Health Association
http://www.apha.org/

Association of Asian Pacific Community Health Organizations (AAPCHO)
http://www.aapcho.org/

Centers for Disease Control and Prevention
http://www.cdc.gov (search for "community health")

Community Health Status Report, U.S. Department of Health and Human Services
http://www.communityhealth.hrsa.gov/

Environmental Protection Agency (EPA)
http://www.epa.gov

Journal of Epidemiology and Community Health
http://jech.bmjjournals.com/

World Health Organization (WHO)
http://www.who.int

WWW Virtual Library on Epidemiology
http://www.epibiostat.ucsf.edu/

WWW Virtual Library on Public Health
http://www.ldb.org.vl/

Part II

What Do Community Health Nurses Do?

3

HEALTH PROMOTION

KEY TERMS

alternative health therapies
continuum model
education
health behavior
health promotion
health promotion model
health protection
health status
Healthy People 2010

integrative model
mutual connectedness model
nutrition
primary prevention
risk factors
secondary prevention
stress
tertiary prevention

HEALTH PROMOTION

A major focus of the community health nurse is health promotion and disease prevention within a larger community setting. This chapter looks at definitions of health, the factors that influence health, and the standards for evaluating health.

KEY POINTS

1. The definition of health has varied through history, but it is agreed that the health functions of the community health nurse consist of the following:

A.   influencing **health behavior**
   i.   People's actions affect their health, either positively or negatively.
   ii. Health behavior has a strong environmental and cultural (family/population) component.

B.   engaging in **health promotion**
   i.   the process of enabling individuals and communities to increase their abilities to control or improve their health
   ii. includes enhancing their physical, social, psychological, and spiritual well-being

C.   assisting in **health protection,** activities that
   i.   help people maintain their current level of health
   ii. prevent disease from occurring
   iii. detect disease early, as through screening
   iv. keep or improve functioning even when disease occurs

2. A number of factors influence **health status.** They include:

A.   individual influences:
   i.   lifestyle (smoking, food choices, alcohol consumption, exercise)
   ii. genetics (family history of illness or wellness)
   iii. behavior (see below)

B.   interpersonal influences:
   i.   social influences such as relationships with family, friends, and people in the community
   ii. work influences, such as availability of work, relationships in the workplace, and the status of the workplace in the community

C.   community influences:
   i.   community resources and programs that are available, and the priority or status that a community gives these influences

D.   environmental influences:
   i.   air and water quality
   ii. presence or absence of pollution
   iii. other environmental hazards, such as toxic sites, noise, vermin

E.   health care system influences:
   i.   a community's perception of the value of available health care
   ii. access (or lack of access) to care
   iii. technology available or not available
   iv. the cost of care

3. Health behavior choices are key to the promotion of health and the prevention of disease. Most crucial areas include:

A. **nutrition**

   i. healthy or unhealthy eating patterns
   ii. adequate or inadequate vitamin or mineral intake
   iii. high-fat or low-fat diet, or vegetarian diet
   iv. nutritional or herbal supplements, or additives
   v. environmental pollutants present in food
   vi. cultural influences about what foods are "good" to eat

B. sleep

   i. Is sleep adequate or inadequate, of good or poor quality?
   ii. How is sleep affected by stress (insomnia, oversleeping)?
   iii. What environmental factors influence sleep (noise, light, temperature, privacy)?
   iv. What cultural components affect sleep patterns (sleep valued, or seen as "wasteful" or "lazy")?

C. physical exercise:

   i. Do individuals exercise? Regularly or not often?
   ii. Is the exercise aerobic or strength-building?
   iii. What cultural determinants affect how individuals feel about exercise?

D. coping with **stress:**

   i. how individuals experience stress connected with illness (such as loss of earning ability, change in family role) and the coping behaviors used
   ii. the cultural determinants of how individuals deal with stress (do cultural expectations forbid discussing the stress or illness, for example, or is a person allowed to talk about the illness, cry, complain, or seek social support?)

4. Another key factor in health promotion and disease prevention functions includes programs such as **Healthy People 2010,** which is part of the U.S. Department of Health and Human Services. Healthy People 2010

A. is used to measure the health of the U.S. population over a 10-year period. The last Healthy People survey was done in 2000.
B. has the major goals of increasing the quality and years of healthy life and eliminating health disparities among different segments of the population.
C. follows a variety of public health indicators, such as:

        i. physical activity and obesity
       ii. drug, alcohol, and tobacco use
      iii. mental health
      iv. incidence of violence and injury
       v. environmental issues
      vi. access to health care

D. seeks information and understanding about the interplay of social and individual responsibility for health and the impact of these factors on public health.

More information about Healthy People 2010 is available at: http:// www.health.gov.healthypeople/

5. A variety of models and theoretical perspectives exist about health and wellness. Most attempt to address the multiple factors that influence health and wellness. Some examples include:

A. **integrative model:** Looks at human health from a biopsychosocial point of view. Key factors that influence health and wellness are seen as emanating from:
        i. the biological sphere (for example, blood sugar levels)
       ii. the psychological sphere (thinking ability, presence of depression)
      iii. the social sphere (socioeconomic status, the availability of social or community support)
      iv. elements are seen as intertwined and interactive

B. **health promotion model**
        i. uses an individual's previous preventive behaviors (such as getting a flu shot or participating in hypertension screening) as a way to evaluate or predict other preventive behaviors
       ii. also understands that these behaviors do not necessarily transfer to all populations

C. **continuum model**
        i. views health as a continuum, from complete health at one extreme, to illness, disability, and death at the other extreme
       ii. focuses on wellness-oriented care and a more holistic perspective, rather than care or definitions of wellness focused only on disease

D. **mutual connectedness model.** Health is defined as a combination of:
        i. an integrated mind, body, and spirit
       ii. a dynamic, responsive, care environment
      iii. the individual's inner relationship with self

6. A variety of **complementary health therapies** are also used in community health nursing.

A. Therapies can include therapeutic touch modalities such as accupressure or massage, and spiritual or religious modalities.

B. Alternative health therapies in community health nursing:

   i. can be used as direct interventions to support healing processes, or to help provide a healing environment

   ii. provide self-help mechanisms that can be taught not only to individuals but also to families or communities

   iii. can be used in primary, secondary, or tertiary situations

C. Examples of complementary therapies include:

   i. mind/body techniques such as relaxation, imagery, meditation

   ii. body techniques such as exercise, yoga, chiropractic, tai chi

   iii. energy techniques such as therapeutic massage, therapeutic touch, shiatsu, accupressure, and reiki reflexology

   iv. spiritual techniques such as faith healing, healing prayer

   v. nutritional therapies such as herbal therapy, macrobiotics, antioxidants

   vi. other therapies such as aromatherapy, pet therapy, music therapy

7. Primary, secondary, and tertiary prevention

A. **Primary prevention:** prevention activities designed to promote health and to prevent diseases and injuries from occurring.

B. **Education** is the key primary health prevention strategy for community health nurses.

C. Effective education programs are interactive, fun, and creative.

D. Primary prevention activities can use a wide variety of media to accomplish different tasks. For example:

   i. storytelling and art, to share how others cope with and succeed in similar situations, and to help people create their own meanings and symbols

   ii. television, available to a wide population, providing opportunities for creative programming

   iii. computers, or other media, to provide interactive learning using visuals and text

E. The cultural characteristics of the target audience should determine which media is preferable, although some media, such as television or art, can often reach across cultural lines.

F. Community health nurses also educate by modeling good health behaviors.

G. **Secondary prevention:** activities focus on detecting disease or illness at its earliest stages, often before there are even clinical signs or symptoms of the illness.

      i.   example: a screening program for tuberculosis
     ii.   Effective secondary prevention relies strongly on the community health nurse's ability to be a sensitive and astute observer during screening, interviewing, history taking, and physical exam.
    iii.   Identification of **risk factors** for a particular illness is also crucial.

H.   **Tertiary prevention:** Prevention activities that occur after a disease or injury is already present, and are focused on preventing or limiting any resulting disabilities.

      i.   Tertiary prevention occurs whether a disease is acute or chronic; degenerative or infectious; or caused by environmental factors.
     ii.   Effective tertiary prevention relies on effective education about medication, follow-up care, and rehabilitation.
    iii.   The focus is not only on physical recovery but also on spiritual and psychological needs during that time.

REVIEW ACTIVITIES

Questions

1. Community health nurses help influence the health of communities through which of the following functions?

   a.   legislating health behavior
   b.   recording health status of individuals in a similar geographic region
   c.   influencing health behavior and engaging in health promotion
   d.   none of the above

2. An example of individual influences on health status would be:

   a.   cigarette smoking
   b.   a parent with adult-onset diabetes
   c.   exposure to toxic substances in the workplace
   d.   all of the above

3. Health promotion activities are designed to:

   a.   prevent people from exposure to germs
   b.   ignore spiritual factors because they can confuse medical issues
   c.   increase communities' control over their health and well-being
   d.   make sure the community health nurse is in charge of health programs

4. Health status is influenced by which of the following:

   a.   lifestyle choices and community resources
   b.   availability of health technology such as diagnostic machines

    c.   presence of toxic environmental conditions

    d.   all of the above

5. The health behavior choices that are essential to promoting health and preventing disease are:

    a.   getting the right kind of food, adequate sleep, physical exercise, and effectively handling stress

    b.   stopping smoking and taking vacations

    c.   making sure that all prescription medications are taken properly and at the right time

    d.   avoiding crowds during flu season

6. Which of the following behaviors are influenced by cultural expectations?

    a.   talking openly about the details of illness

    b.   deciding whether to "feed a cold" or "starve a fever"

    c.   taking herbal supplements to boost the immune system

    d.   all of the above

7. Healthy People 2010 is designed to:

    a.   track health care trends so that future insurance liabilities can be anticipated, especially for poor and urban populations

    b.   show that social factors have little or no impact on individual and community health

    c.   follow health indicators such as activity, substance use, mental health, and environmental issues

    d.   show that access to health care in the United States is adequate for all populations

8. Integrative models of human health see health factors as:

    a.   derived solely from physical phenomena

    b.   intertwined and interactive, with multiple components such as physical, psychological, and social

    c.   generally being attributable to psychological problems in individuals

    d.   effective only when combined and integrated with alternative therapies

9. An example of the continuum model of health and wellness would be:

    a.   a person is either well or not, and the emphasis is on continuously and aggressively treating people who are ill

    b.   predicting that a person will most likely continue good health practices, based on her or his health practices in the past, such as getting flu shots

    c.   using acupuncture and therapeutic touch to cure disease instead of traditional medical therapies

    d.   none of the above

10. A key component of primary prevention strategies is:

  a. aggressive intervention
  b. detection
  c. culture
  d. education

11. An example of a secondary prevention strategy would be:

  a. screening for breast cancer in women who have no symptoms
  b. using pain control medications for terminal cancer patients
  c. educating teenagers about using condoms to prevent the spread of STDs
  d. none of the above

Critical-Thinking Questions

1. How does the community health nurse influence health behavior and assist in health protection for people in communities? What are the advantages and disadvantages of these functions?

2. How do you deal with illness-related stress? Are you more like or unlike your family or culture? Compare your coping behaviors with those of someone you know well. How are the behaviors alike and different? What would a community health nurse need to know to be most helpful to you?

3. Which health model—integrative, health promotion, continuum, or mutual connectedness—do you think is most useful in dealing with a client population? Why or why not? Which model most closely resembles your approach?

4. What complementary therapies are you familiar with? How have you seen them used in client care? Are they effective or not?

5. Give an example of primary, secondary, and tertiary prevention strategies for tuberculosis.

Discussion Questions

1. Individual, interpersonal, community, and environmental influences all affect the health status of a community. For a community you are involved in, name two key factors in each area. For your community, which factors have the most effect? The least?

2. Healthy People 2010 follows a variety of health indicators such as physical activity and obesity; drug, alcohol, and tobacco use; mental health; incidence of violence and injury; environmental issues; and access to health care. For a population in your community, which of these indicators do you think has the greatest impact on health and wellness?

3. What media are used in your community to promote health and prevent illness or disease? Give three examples and discuss how effective they are for their target audience.

References

Ahronheim, J. C. (2000). *Ethics in clinical practice* (2nd ed.). Gaithersburg, MD: Aspen.

Clark, C. C. (Ed.). (1999). *Encyclopedia of complementary health care practice*. New York: Springer.

Diamond, B. (1998). *The legal aspects of complementary therapy practice: A guide for health care professionals*. New York: Churchill-Livingstone.

Fontaine, K. L. (2000). *Healing practices: Alternative therapies for nursing*. Upper Saddle River, NJ: Prentice-Hall.

Freeman, L. W. (2001). *Mosby's complementary and alternative medicine: A research-based approach*. St. Louis, MO: Mosby.

Hitchcock, J., Schubert, P., & Thomas, S. (1999). *Community health nursing: Caring in action*. Clifton Park, NY: Delmar Learning.

Jordan, M. L., & Delunas, L. R. (2001). Quality of life and patterns of nontraditional therapy use by patients with cancer. *Oncol Nurs Forum, 28*(7), 1107–1113.

Keegan, L. (1998). Alternative and complementary therapies. *Nursing 98, 28*(4), 50–53.

Richardson, J., Jones, C., & Pilkington, K. (2001). Complementary therapies: What is the evidence for their use? *Prof Nurs, 17*(2), 96–99.

White, L. (2001). *Foundations of nursing: Caring for the whole person.* Clifton Park, NY: Delmar Learning.

Willich, S. W., & Elm, S. (2001). *Medical challenges for the new millennium: An interdisciplinary task.* Dordrecht, the Netherlands: Kluwer Academic Publishers.

Web Sites

Alternative Health News Online
http://www.altmedicine.com/

Alternative Medicine Homepage
http://www.pitt.edu/~cbw.altm.html

Centers for Disease Control and Prevention (causes of death)
http://www.cdc.gov/

Healthy People 2010
http://www.health.gov.healthypeople/

National Library of Medicine
http://www.nlm.nih.gov

Psychoneuroimmunology Research Society
http://www.pnirs.org/

THE ROLE OF THE NURSE

advocate
case manager
clinician
collaborator
consultant
counselor

educator
hospice care
parish health nurse
researcher
self-care
self-determination

INTRODUCTION

Nurses working in a community setting adopt a number of different roles: advocate, collaborator, consultant, counselor, and more. The community health nurse must be able to perform multiple role functions due to the focus on aggregate populations rather than individuals This chapter examines the varied roles that a community health nurse adopts and why each of these roles is important.

KEY POINTS

1. **Clinician:** The community health nurse acts as a clinician, for example, when screening people at a neighborhood clinic for immunization status.

Focus is not on the one-on-one, clinician role seen in individual medicine but on the health of individuals in the larger context of the community or society.

   A.   Goals for the nurse as clinician are to reduce disease, discomfort, disability, and premature death for the total community.

   B.   The number of nurses in this role in the community will increase significantly in the future.

   C.   This role can be filled by nurses who are generalists or specialists.

2. Advocate: The community health nurse acts as advocate for a community or group.

   A.   The nurse speaks or acts for those who may not be able to speak or act for themselves, due to:

       i.   lack of knowledge
      ii.   inability to articulate needs
    iii.   fear
    iv.   perceived lack of power
     v.   physical or mental disability

   B.   In this role a community health nurse might speak to a city council about the medication and follow-up needs of the homeless population.

   C.   Community health nurses are often best equipped to help people negotiate the complexities of the current medical system.

   D.   Community health nurses have broad exposure to social situations and are closely tied to family and community. As a result they can more effectively advocate for a group.

   E.   Community health nurse advocates:

       i.   promote **self-care**—people's ability to be active participants in their own health care
      ii.   support **self-determination**—the right people have to make the choices that are best for themselves or their community

3. Collaborator: The community health nurse works with people in the community toward a common goal.

   A.   To collaborate, or to work together, bring together the strengths and resources of all the people involved. For example, a community health nurse in this role might:

       i.   work together with neighborhood AIDS activists to strategize how to write, produce, and distribute posters telling about a new needle exchange program
      ii.   help get this information to the local media

B. Effective collaboration relies on joint or shared decision making that reflects the respect all parties have for one another.
C. Effective collaboration also requires cooperation, effective communication, and problem-solving skills.
D. Community health nurses may collaborate with:

   i. people in the community
   ii. other members of the health care team
   iii. political, religious, judicial, volunteer, social service, and other community organizations

4. **Consultant:** The community health nurse also acts as a consultant, providing information, helping clients understand, and assisting in decision making and choosing actions that are most appropriate or beneficial.

A. In this role, for example, a community health nurse could provide information on health care and third-party payers to elderly people on limited incomes, so they can decide which supplemental insurance is best for their needs.
B. Effective consulting can consist of:

   i. acting as a catalyst to help bring about change
   ii. helping people understand processes and actions, to learn about how they make decisions
   iii. filling the role of information providers/experts and teachers

C. The task of the consultant is not to make decisions for people but to help them make good decisions for themselves by providing information or strategies that make success possible.
D. The best consulting relationships are collaborative—with both nurse and clients active and responsible. However, clients need to make the final decision.

5. **Counselor:** The community health nurse's roles may also include counselor.

A. A counselor helps people choose the most appropriate solutions or options, not by deciding for them, but by strengthening and guiding people's own decision-making skills or processes.
B. In this role, a community health nurse could help a culturally diverse neighborhood group explore their feelings about conflict and conflict resolution.
C. Key tasks for the counseling role include listening, and providing feedback and information.
D. Counseling may use exploration of feelings and attitudes to help people understand themselves and their decision making more completely.

E.   The counseling role is often combined with other roles such as consulting or educating.

6. **Educator:** The community health nurse may act as an educator.

A.   Educators provide people with information, knowledge, or skills that they need to make appropriate choices or decisions.
B.   For example, a community health nurse educator could provide reliable information about birth control methods, reliability, and side effects to teens and young adults.
C.   Key tasks for the educator include:

   i.   enabling clients to make informed decisions about personal, family, or community health practices and lifestyle choices, by providing knowledge and skills
   ii. identifying populations at risk and implementing effective teaching strategies for these groups, including participatory and other culturally appropriate methods
   iii. exploring strategies for ongoing learning in the population

D.   Culturally sensitive teaching guidelines include the following:

   i.   Make sure you know the client's cultural background.
   ii. Be alert for behaviors or practices that differ from what you perceive as "normal."
   iii. Be aware that family dynamics are different in different cultures: observe the interactions of family members to determine roles, dominance, who should be included in conversations or decisions, and the like.
   iv. Check that the client understands you; do not talk down to him or her, but avoid using complex medical terms or jargon.
   v.   Make sure that the client understands your nonverbal language, and that you understand the client's (in many cultures, for example, a nod of the head does not always mean "yes").

7. **Researcher:** The community health nurse may act as a researcher, gathering data of different types for different purposes.

A.   Tasks of the researcher can include:

   i.   identifying problems
   ii. working with data (collecting, analyzing, interpreting)
   iii. conducting research (designing, evaluating)

B.   A reliable research foundation allows nurses to anticipate potential health problems for a population and to promote interventions based on reliable data.

C. A community health nurse involved in this type of work must remain up-to-date on current research and search for ways to apply research to practice.

8. Case Manager: The community health nurse may (and often does) act as a case manager.

A. Case management involves the complex task of coordinating care in a system that is made up of many different programs, which have different policies, services, and missions.
B. For example, a community health nurse acting as a case manager could coordinate the varied and sometimes specialized levels of physical and mental health care for residents of a group home for developmentally disabled adults.
C. Key tasks are to avoid gaps in service and breakdown in the care system, especially for more vulnerable populations who cannot manage or control their own care.
D. Case management is particularly effective for community health settings and for populations with long-term care needs:

    i. elderly
    ii. chronically ill
    iii. mentally or physically disabled
    iv. homeless
    v. nursing home residents
    vi. members of other high-risk groups

E. Case management can also be used to control costs associated with inefficient use, or lack of coordination, of available resources.

9. Community health and home health nursing are similar in that both:

A. care for clients in a variety of settings
B. practice independently outside institutions
C. include clients as active participants in care decisions
D. include families in client care
E. help organize and provide services
F. have broad goals of promoting, maintaining, and restoring health

10. Community health and home health nursing are different in these ways:

A. Community health nursing focuses on populations while home health focuses on individuals or families.
B. Community health nursing cases are received from the community while home health nursing cases are referred by a physician or other agency.

C.   Community health nursing intervention is continuous while home health nursing is as needed.

D.   Community health nursing has a strong emphasis on primary prevention and wellness. Home health nursing's first emphasis is responding to or treating illness, followed by secondary and tertiary prevention, and rehabilitation.

E.   Community health nursing becomes involved in the community through assessing risk potential and using primarily social diagnoses; home health nursing uses the medical diagnosis model as its entry point.

11. Hospice care

A.   Hospice care is a coordinated program of palliative services, and another key setting for community health nurse.

B.   Key role of the community health nurse includes:

  i.   working as part of an interdisciplinary team
  ii. helping the client and family maintain the client's dignity and comfort
  iii. promoting appropriate palliative care for the client
  iv. identifying and addressing caregiver, family, or community needs

C.   Key nursing tasks include:

  i.   providing care skills in a home or other setting
  ii. knowing community resources
  iii. ability to work as part of a multidisciplinary, diverse care team
  iv. ability to balance needs of the client and family and personal needs and self-care

12. End-of-Life Care

A.   Health care professionals should not impose their own opinion on end-of-life decisions made by clients.

B.   Health care professionals can decline to participate in care (ask for a different assignment) if they find care requested by the client objectionable.

C.   If a client has refused specific care (for example, chemotherapy), comfort measures must continue, including the treatment of pain.

D.   Nurses should be aware of their institution's or agency's policies and procedures that are to be followed for end-of-life care, particularly when treatment is refused or life support is withdrawn. These can include:

       i. client's right to refuse
      ii. documentation of refusal
     iii. pain control
     iv. definition of terms such as Do Not Resuscitate (DNR)
      v. management of client comfort
     vi. nurse's role in caring for clients who refuse treatment or have treatment withheld

E. DNR orders must follow appropriate protocol. Requirements generally include:

      i. order must be in writing and must be renewed
      ii. order must be given in person rather than by phone
     iii. client must be resuscitated if no DNR exists
     iv. DNR is clearly defined so other treatments (such as pain alleviation) can continue if needed

F. The community health nurse may institute a community-based DNR program for terminally ill clients in the community, particularly those in hospice, who do not wish to be resuscitated. Clients are typically identified by a special wristband. In some communities, this is done in collaboration with:

      i. physicians who write the order
      ii. the emergency medical system, which may be called for the client if breathing or heart beat ceases and family members panic
     iii. the local emergency department, to which a client may be taken

13. Parish Health Nursing

A. The **parish health nurse** provides holistic nursing services, as part of a pastoral or ministerial team, to the members of a faith community or congregation.
B. This role is adapted from historical religion-based models.
C. Key tasks are that the nurse integrates theological, psychological, sociological, and physiological perspectives about health and healing with the beliefs and culture of the congregation. In this role, the nurse:

      i. uses faith and support networks of religious congregations to meet health promotion and disease prevention needs of its members
      ii. identifies a population by its value orientation, spiritual needs and direction, and associations of community and culture
     iii. does not provide invasive treatments but gives a framework to help group members improve or maintain health

REVIEW ACTIVITIES

Questions

1. The community health nurse acting in the role of clinician would be most likely to:
   a. work to articulate the special needs of a population such as homeless people
   b. focus on reducing the incidence of disease in a population
   c. address the spiritual needs of a group without performing any screening or treatments
   d. coordinate the various components of care in different areas of the health system

2. The community health nurse acting in the role of advocate would be most likely to promote:
   a. self-care and self-determination for the population
   b. telling people in a community that the medical experts know what is best for them
   c. smoking cessation
   d. that health care options should be pursued without the influence of friends or family

3. An example of collaboration between a community health nurse and a population would be:
   a. the nurse providing educational pamphlets about drug and alcohol use
   b. shared decision making between the nurse, the community, and a local hospital about the hours of operation and staffing for a community health center
   c. helping people in the community explore feelings about the death of a community resident
   d. none of the above

4. Nurses acting as researchers can help communities by:
   a. educating the community about how care can be coordinated
   b. ignoring data generated by research because these data have no connection with the provision of quality care
   c. showing how research is culturally biased
   d. using reliable data to anticipate health problems and promote interventions based on these data

5. The advantage of a community health nurse acting as a case manager includes:

a. managing complex tasks and coordinating care in a multifunction system
b. coordinating care needs for special populations
c. avoiding breakdown or gaps in care for vulnerable populations or those with long-term needs
d. all of the above

6. Which of the following tasks would be appropriate for a community health nurse acting as a counselor?
a. motivating people to be politically active
b. encouraging people to be passive so as not to upset the decision makers
c. listening and providing feedback and information
d. showing people how exploring feelings and attitudes is not important for meeting health care needs

7. Which of the following is *not* a role for the community health nurse providing hospice or end-of-life care?
a. providing resources for caregivers to prevent burnout
b. ensuring that the client is given every reasonable chance to extend life and is encouraged to not give up too easily
c. working as part of a multidisciplinary team to meet client, family, and community needs
d. promoting and coordinating palliative care and services

8. Which of the following is true about end-of-life care?
a. The nurse has no role in end-of-life care, as care is turned over to the family.
b. The nurse must always continue to provide care for a client, even when the family makes end-of-life decisions that the nurse disagrees with.
c. Decisions to resuscitate a client do not need to be in writing but can be started verbally by a family member or close friend.
d. Care such as pain management continues even if a client has refused life-prolonging treatment.

9. Which of the following is true about the role of a parish health nurse?
a. The nurse provides any medical treatments necessary to cure disease and promote health.
b. The nurse uses a religious congregation's faith and support networks to promote health and prevent disease.
c. The nurse takes the place of the ministerial team.
d. The nurse does not attempt to integrate theological perspectives about health and well-being.

Critical-Thinking Questions

1. Describe how the roles of the community health nurse as researcher and as educator might overlap.

2. How are the roles of consultant and educator alike? What is a key difference?

3. How are community health nursing and home health nursing alike? Different?

Discussion Questions

1. What types of self-care or self-determination options are available for people in your community? Name the role that community health nurses play, if any.

2. Identify examples in your community in which nurses act as:
   • clinicians
   • advocates
   • consultants
   • counselors
   • educators
   • researchers
   • case managers

   Do some nurses have multiple roles? Give an example.

3. What hospice care is available in your community? How do people usually find out about these services?

4. Think about the religious communities or congregations in your area. Do any of them have a parish health nurse as part of their pastoral or ministerial team? How could religious communities or congregations in your area benefit from having a parish health nurse?

References

American Nurses Association. (1986a). *Standards of community health nursing practice*. Kansas City, MO. American Nurses Association.

American Nurses Association. (1986b). *Standards of home health nursing practice*. Kansas City, MO: American Nurses Association.

American Nurses Association. (1986c). *Standards and scope of hospice nursing practice*. Kansas City, MO: American Nurses Association.

Drennan, V., & Williams, G. (2001). An assessment of dual-role primary care nurses in the inner city. *Br J Community Nurs, 6*(7), 336–341.

Gamlin, R. (2001). Ethical issues in palliative care. *Int J Palliative Nurs, 7*(7), 360.

Huston, C. J. (2001). The role of the case manager in a disease management program. *Lippincott Case Manage, 6*(5), 222–227.

McGovern, M. (2001). A nurse-led service to provide palliative care in the community. *Prof Nurse, 17*(2), 127–128.

Rodgers, B. (2000). Coordination of care: The lived experience of the visiting nurse. *Home Health Care Nurse, 18*(5), 301–307.

Water, C. M. (2000). End of life care directives among African Americans: Lesssons learned: A need for community centered discussions and education. *Journal of Community Health Nursing, 17*(1), 25–37.

Whiley, K. (2001). The nurse manager's role in creating a healthy work environment. *AACN Clin Issues Adv Pract Acute Crit Care, 12*(3), 356–365.

Web Sites

Homecare Online: National Association for Home Care
http://www.nahc.org

Hospice and Palliative Care Nurses Association
http://www.hpna.org/

Hospice Foundation of America
http://www.hospicefoundation.org

Journal of Community Health Nursing (online version)
http://www.catchword.com/

National Hospice and Palliative Care Organization
http://www.nhpco.org/

National Hospice Foundation
http://www.hospiceinfo.org/

National Institute of Nursing Research
http://www.nih.gov/ninr/

National League for Nursing
http://www.nln.org

Partnership for Caring: America's Voices for the Dying (formerly Choices in Dying)
http://www.partnershipforcaring.org/

Visiting Nurses Association of America (VNAA)
http://www.vnaa.org

EPIDEMIOLOGY

agent
analytical study
attack rate
case control study
case fatality rate
case study
cause-specific death rate
chemical agent
cohort study
correlation study
cross-sectional survey
demography
descriptive study
environment
epidemiology
epidemiological study
etiology
fetal death rate
host
human ecology
incidence rate

infectious agent
interrelationships
intervention study
observational study
maternal mortality rate
morbidity rate
mortality rate
natural history of disease
nutritive agent
perinatal mortality rate
physical agent
prevention trials
prevalence rate
primary prevention
prospective study
relative risk
retrospective study
secondary prevention
tertiary prevention
therapeutic trials
vital statistics

INTRODUCTION

Community health nurses use epidemiology as a tool to identify vulnerable populations; possible causes, and the risk factors that may be contributing to a disease or injury. This chapter introduces and discusses the uses, purposes, and limitations of epidemiology.

KEY POINTS

1. **Epidemiology** is a population-focused, applied science that uses research and statistical data collection methods to discover:

   A. which populations are affected by disease or injury
   B. how often these conditions occur in the population
   C. the risk factors or causal factors that may be contributing to these conditions

2. Using epidemiology can also lead community health nurses to the possible **etiology** (cause) of health problems in a population or area.

3. Community health is made up of three applied sciences: epidemiology, human ecology, and demography:

   A. epidemiology: studies a broad spectrum of communicable and chronic diseases, injury control, nutrition, and violence
   B. **human ecology:** the interrelationship between people and their environments
   C. **demography:** measurements of population characteristics, such as births, deaths, age distribution, and other vital statistics

4. An epidemiological approach assumes that disease, injury, and health do not occur randomly. A key function of the epidemiological approach is to find the etiology (cause) of the disease or risk factor.

5. Epidemiologists systematically study three elements to determine the etiology of health problems in a population: agent, host, and environment:

   A. **agent:** a toxic substance, microorganism, or environmental factor that must be present or absent for the problem to occur. Agents can be classified as:

      i. **infectious agent:** bacteria, viruses, fungi, metazoa, or protozoa

    ii. **physical agent:** excessive exposure to physical elements such as
         sun or radiation; mechanical such as carpal tunnel or overuse
         syndrome
    iii. **chemical agent:**
         a. poisons such as insecticides, paints, poisonous plants, or ani-
             mals
         b. caustic substances such as lye
         c. carbon monoxide
         d. overdoses of otherwise nonpoisonous substances such as pre-
             scription or over-the-counter medications
         e. allergens such as poison ivy, tree pollen, or certain foods or
             medications
    iv. **nutritive agent:** the lack of needed substances, such as vitamins,
         minerals, or protein; or the excess of a particular substance, such
         as a diet with high fat or salt content

  B. **host:** the person or population on which the agent acts. Hosts are
      affected by

      i. demographic agents such as age, ethnicity, and socioeconomic
          status
      ii. genetic factors
  C. **environment:** factors outside the host that are associated with develop-
      ment of disease, disorder, or injury. Environmental factors can include:

      i.   geographical factors
      ii. occupational factors
      iii. personal factors such as lifestyle or activity level

6. Epidemiologists also look closely at the interactions and **interrelationships**
   among agent, host, and environment elements.

7. The purpose of an epidemiological study is to understand the **natural history of a disease,** the unaltered course that a disease would follow if there
   were no interventions such as therapy or lifestyle changes.

  A. Knowing the natural history of a disease can lead to the development
      of prevention strategies or therapeutic interventions.
  B. Community health nurses use this key concept in educating people
      about diseases.

8. Prevention is a key concept in epidemiology. There are three levels of prevention: primary, secondary, and tertiary.

  A. **Primary prevention:**
      i. strategies or interventions to foster health and wellness before
          disease or symptoms develop

      ii. can include education, regulation, and immunization.

  B. **Secondary prevention:**

      i. strategies that target early diagnosis and treatment, focusing on detecting and treating disease before disability or impairment occurs

      ii. can include screening programs, and early diagnosis and appropriate treatment for diseases such as heart disease and tuberculosis, before these conditions become severe

  C. **Tertiary prevention:** strategies and activities to limit disability once disease develops

9. **Epidemiological studies** are used to examine what kind of health problems occur in populations, how widely occurring they are, and what causes them. Types of epidemiological studies include:

  A. **Observational studies:** nonexperimental studies that describe, compare, and explain the occurrence of disease or injury in a population.

  B. Observational studies can be **descriptive studies** of epidemiology. Types of descriptive studies include:

      i. **correlation study:** allows assessment of a disease by examining its occurrence as related to risk factors.

      ii. **cross-sectional survey:** allows assessment of a representative group (cross-section) of a population.

      iii. **case study** or history: allows assessment of detailed health information about individuals or groups within a population.

  C. Observational studies can also be **analytical studies,** which seek to compare and study possible associations and causal relationships. Analytical observational studies include:

      i. **case control** or **retrospective study:**
        a. assesses a group of individuals after a disease or incident has occurred in comparison to a similar unaffected group
        b. examines possible risk factors that might be associated with the disease or incident

      ii. **cohort** or **prospective study:**
        a. assesses a group of individuals who do not have the disease being studied
        b. follows the group into the future to determine the effect of risk factors on disease development

  D. **Intervention studies:** The second type of epidemiological study is experimental and requires altering the behavior of the participants rather than just observing the behavior. These studies include:

      i. **prevention trials:** to test interventions

ii. **therapeutic trials:** in which an experimental group receives a drug or procedure and is then compared to a control group, which does not receive the drug or procedure

10. Epidemiological measurements allow comparison of disease occurrences between groups. The most commonly used measurements are:

A. **prevalence rate:** the proportion of the population that has the disease at any one time
B. **incidence rate:** the rate of change from people who do not have disease to having disease. This rate reflects new cases of a disease or condition during a specified time.
C. **morbidity rate:** the incidence of nonfatal cases in the total at-risk population during a specified time
D. **attack rate:** the occurrence of the disease or condition among a particular at-risk population, often due to a specific exposure. The attack rate is calculated only for a limited time
E. **mortality rate:** the death rate. The mortality rate can reflect both incidence and prevalence
F. **case fatality rate:** the number of deaths from a specific disease

11. Vital statistics are the result of systematic registration of vital events such as births, deaths, and health events. They are used to examine incidence and prevalence in various populations. Key vital statistics are:

A. **cause-specific death rate:** the number of deaths due to a given cause in a year
B. **maternal mortality rate:** the number of maternal deaths at the time of birth or shortly thereafter
C. **fetal death rate:** the number of fetal deaths in one year
D. **perinatal mortality rate:** the number of deaths in infants less than 7 days old

12. Relative risk indicates the likelihood of an exposed group developing a disease relative to those who are not exposed.

13. Uses of the epidemiological approach in community health nursing:

A. For disease and health status surveillance, epidemiological approach provides:
i. a systematic count of disease frequency
ii. a search for etiology, to identify connections between demographics or environmental characteristics of a community and the incidence of disease

B. For future health planning and evaluating the effectiveness of education and other programs in the community.

REVIEW ACTIVITIES

Questions

1. Which of the following statements best describes the term *epidemiology*?
    a. applied science that uses surveys to track communicable diseases (spread from person to person)
    b. applied science that uses research and statistics to find out about how disease affects populations and the reasons disease occurs
    c. applied science whose sole function is to find the etiology of all diseases
    d. applied science that uses correlation studies to determine the appropriate tertiary prevention strategies for a community

2. Community health is made up of which of the following?
    a. epidemiology, parasitology, and correlation studies
    b. etiology studies, prevention, and demographics
    c. epidemiology, human ecology, and demography
    d. infectious agents, natural history of a disease, and demography

3. Which of the following factors can contribute to a person being a host?
    a. exposure to physical, chemical, or nutritive agents
    b. being young or old
    c. poverty
    d. all of the above

4. Which of the following statements about the natural history of a disease is correct?
    a. It has nothing to do with epidemiological studies.
    b. Using this method works only for communicable diseases.
    c. Following the course the disease would take if there were no interventions can lead to developing strategies or therapeutic interventions.
    d. None of the above

5. A community health nurse is participating in an analytic study of people who are at risk for developing diabetes. Studies of this type are classified as:
    a. retrospective
    b. concurrent
    c. cross-sectional
    d. prospective

6. A community health nurse is participating in an analytic study of people who developed melanoma following frequent visits to tanning salons. Studies of this type are classified as:
    a. retrospective
    b. concurrent
    c. cross-sectional
    d. prospective

7. Which of the following characteristics apply to intervention studies?
    a. They do not require altering the behavior of study subjects, only observing them.
    b. They include prevention or therapeutic trials.
    c. They follow the group being studied into the future to determine risk factors.
    d. They are the same as correlation studies.

8. Which statement most accurately reflects prevalence rate and incidence rate?
    a. There is no difference; they mean the same thing.
    b. Prevalence rate indicates the rate of change from people who do not have the disease, to their having it.
    c. Both cover unspecified, unlimited periods of time.
    d. Incidence rate reflects new cases of a disease during a specified time.

9. Which of the following are considered key vital statistics?
    a. attack rate and morbidity rate
    b. incidence and prevalence rate
    c. maternal mortality rate and fetal death rate
    d. relative risk

Critical-Thinking Questions

1. A community health nurse is concerned about the increased number of persons who have reported symptoms of nausea, vomiting, and diarrhea after eating in a particular restaurant. What is the first step the nurse should take? Why?

2. A community health nurse is participating in an analytical epidemiological study of a specific health problem and is asked to identify cohorts of those affected by the health problem. If those with the health problem being studied are from 30 to 40 years of age and live in a particular geographic community, what characteristics would the cohorts have?

Discussion Questions

1. What are the vital statistics for your community, for example, maternal mortality rate, fetal death rate, perinatal mortality rate? Do they vary by geographic location? By ethnicity? By socioeconomic status? Where do you go in your community to find these data?

2. What kinds of epidemiological studies have been performed in your community in the past five years? Do you know what kind of studies they were (descriptive, analytical, intervention?) How were they conducted? What were the results? In your community, what groups or organizations are most involved in conducting epidemiological studies?

References

Fawcett, J., & Gigliotti, E. (2001). Using conceptual models of nursing to guide nursing research: The case of the Neuman systems model. *Nurs Sci Q, 14*(4), 339–345.

FitzGerald, M., McCutcheon, H., Court, A., & Athanasiadis, K. (2001). Engaging nurses in clinical research. *Nurs Times, 97*(37), 38–39.

Gordes, L. (2000). *Epidemiology*. Philadelphia: W. B. Saunders.

Hitchcock, J., Schubert, P., & Thomas, S. (1999). *Community health nursing: Caring in action*. Clifton Park, NY: Delmar Learning.

Lilenfeld, D., & Stolley, P. (1994). *Foundations of epidemiology*. New York: Oxford University Press.

McCormack, D., & MacIntosh, J. (2001). Research with homeless people uncovers a model of health. *West J Nurs Res, 23*(7), 698–713.

Rothman, K. (Ed.). (1998). *Modern epidemiology*. Philadelphia: Lippincott, Williams & Wilkins.

Swanson, J. M., & Nies, M. (Eds.). (1997). *Community health nursing: Promoting the health of aggregates.* Philadelphia: Saunders.

Web Sites

American Journal of Epidemiology
http://aje.oupjournals.org/

Centers for Disease Control and Prevention, Epidemiology Program Office
http://www.cdc.gov/epo/

Epidemiology. The Official Journal of the International Society for Environmental Epidemiology
http://www.epidem.com/

Epidemiology Supercourse
http://www.pitt.edu/~super1/

Epidemiology for the uninitiated
http://www.burj.com/epidem/epid.html

World Wide Web Virtual Library: Epidemiology
http://www.epibiostat.ucsf.edu/epidem/epidem.html

6

COMMUNITY ASSESSMENT

community
community assessment
community assessment process
community assessment tools
community capacity
community competence

community of interest
multicultural factors
process
status
structure

INTRODUCTION

Community health nurses are often called upon to assess a community or population in order to identify and define problems and strengths. This chapter introduces community assessment, and reviews the steps of a community assessment and the tools nurses use in performing a community assessment.

KEY POINTS

1. A core task of community health nursing practice is for the community health nurse to identify problems as well as address the nature of the problems.

2. Definitions of community can differ. The term **community** can include:

   A. groups of diverse or similar people living in one geographic location
   B. an interactive link of families, friends, and organizations

C. systems or groups bound by shared needs and interests

3. The term **community of interest** is often used by community health nurses to describe groups of people who share beliefs, values, or interests, but who may not live in the same geographic area.

4. Some communities are not homogeneous and may have conflicting interests or needs.

5. The following three dimensions need to be included in any definition of community:

A. **status:** information about morbidity and mortality, life expectancy, crime rates, and education
B. **structure:** the socioeconomic, age, gender, and ethnic distribution as well as resources available
C. **process:** how the community operates; how it functions as a whole to solve problems
D. Process also includes the concept of **community competence,** or the community's ability to:
   i. identify needs effectively
   ii. achieve working consensus on issues
   iii. agree on ways to implement goals
   iv. work together to implement desired actions

6. Community capacity is defined as the resources, strengths, and abilities the community brings to work on a particular issue. Community capacity builds on community competence.

7. Community participation in community assessment is essential. The community health nurse has a key role in making sure that community participation processes truly include and empower members of the community, rather than just directing or co-opting them.

8. Community assessment is the process of examining a community's characteristics, assets and resources, liabilities, and needs, in collaboration with the community, to develop strategies that improve health and quality of life for the community.

9. The **community assessment process** involves the following steps:

A. Identify available resources—for example, time and money to conduct the assessment; skills and time requirements of team members.

B. Establish project team (people to do the assessment) and steering committee (people who oversee the project and provide advice or guidance).
C. Develop research plan and time frame to help the assessment stay on track and on schedule.
D. Collect and analyze information that already exists and is available to avoid reinventing the wheel (for example, literature reviews for similar projects, similar data collected in other studies or by government agencies).
E. Complete community research using surveys, interviews, group discussions, and so on.
F. Analyze results, looking closely at the data to determine what they mean. Analysis should always be linked to the original purpose of the assessment.
G. Report back to the community using reports, meetings, mass media, displays in frequented areas, or presentations.
H. Set priorities for action. Setting priorities depends on the needs present, the number of people affected, the consequences of needs not being met, whether needs might be met in other ways, and available resources.
I. Determine the best way to address the needs that were identified: it is essential that the community have input in this decision.
J. Plan and implement the strategies that are selected.

10. **Community assessment tools** include the following:

A. literature review
B. national and local policy documents
C. demographic and epidemiological data
D. focus groups
E. previously conducted community surveys
F. participant observation
G. community leaders or experts
H. surveys of community members

11. **Multicultural factors** that need to be taken into account in assessing communities include differences in:

A. communication: for example, whether the culture values direct, explicit communication or prefers to communicate indirectly or implicitly
B. personal space
    i. the amount of space required between people so that they feel comfortable and not that their space is being invaded

      ii. This space is often defined differently in various cultures, or differently within the same culture, depending on who is talking, the gender of those involved, whether it is a public or private conversation, and so forth.

  C. reactions to authority: for example, whether cultural rules prohibit speaking openly to persons in authority, or saying what they want to hear

  D. social organization: the strength or flexibility of familial and acquaintance ties

  E. perception of time:

      i. Does the culture perceive punctuality and time efficiency as important or polite?

      ii. Is time perceived as less important than relationships and interaction?

12. It is essential for community health nurses to be familiar with multicultural characteristics of the communities they work with, for these reasons:

  A. Different cultural practices can impact whether or not prevention or treatment is successful.

  B. Different races or ethnic groups can have different reactions to certain drugs or treatment regimens.

REVIEW ACTIVITIES

Questions

1. Which of the following statements best describes a community?
  a. people living in a particular geographic location
  b. organizations, family groups, or friend groups that interact
  c. groups that have common interests or needs
  d. all of the above

2. A community of interest could be described as:
  a. people who live in the same geographic area and share common interests
  b. people who share beliefs, values, or interests but not a geographic location
  c. people with the ability to identify their own needs
  d. people who have the same life expectancy

3. A community that is described as having community competence has which of the following characteristics?

    a. the ability to perform their own cross-sectional epidemiological studies
    b. the ability to delegate any community processes to an outside expert such as a community health nurse
    c. the ability to identify their needs, achieve consensus, and plan and implement goals
    d. the ability to predict morbidity and mortality rates for the population or geographic area

4. The key role for the community health nurse in dealing with communities is to:

    a. make sure that people in the community are empowered and able to participate
    b. provide incentives for community members to follow the protocols of any study or drug trial
    c. establish project teams that will collect and analyze data
    d. closely direct community members so that the community assessments are done appropriately

5. Which of the following is *not* a part of the community assessment process?

    a. identifying available resources such as time, money, and team skills
    b. collecting and analyzing information
    c. withholding results from the community until they can be statistically confirmed, to avoid alarming people
    d. setting action priorities based on the needs of the community and available resources

6. Which of the following describes a valid way to collect data for a community assessment?

    a. using a library database to conduct a literature review
    b. reading government documents to find if similar data have already been collected
    c. using surveys or questionnaires to gather information from members of the community
    d. all of the above

7. A younger community member's reluctance to speak to an older community health nurse might be due to a difference in cultural perception about:

    a. personal space
    b. honesty
    c. authority
    d. perception of time

8. Cultural differences in perceptions about time might be shown as:
   a. engaging in several minutes of casual conversation before talking with the nurse about a health issue
   b. always arriving at appointment times 15 minutes earlier than the scheduled time
   c. arriving at an appointment a half hour later than the scheduled time
   d. all of the above

Critical-Thinking Questions

1. A community health nurse is attempting to conduct a community assessment for a neighborhood group with a high incidence of teenage pregnancy and STDs. Although the teenagers take the surveys and say they will fill them out, they do not. Or if they do fill them out, they provide little or no information about sexual activity. What does this nurse need to understand about the culture of this group?

2. What is the distance of your personal space, in inches? How does this space differ for the different people in your lives? Does it differ from that of others in your family or community? What happens when someone enters your personal space without your permission?

Discussion Questions

1. For the community in which you live or work, define its status, structure, and process. Which of these dimensions are most important in how you perceive your community?

2. Pick a community that you have worked with. How would you describe that community's competence? What abilities are present? Absent?

References

Anderson, P. M., Loudon, R. F., Greenfield, S. M., & Gill, P. S. (2001). Nursing in a diverse community: A narrative view. *Nurse Educ Today, 21*(6), 423–433.

Huff, R. M., & Kline, M. V. (Eds.). (1999). *Promoting health in multicultural populations: A handbook for practitioners.* Thousand Oaks, CA: Sage.

Kar, S. B., et al. (Eds.). (2000). *Health communication: A multicultural perspective.* Thousand Oaks, CA: Sage.

Kim-Godwin, Y. S., Clarke, P. N., & Barton, L. J. (2001). A model for the delivery of culturally competent community care. *Adv Nurs, 35*(6), 918–925.

King, N., & Henderson, G. (Eds.). (1999). *Beyond regulations: Ethics in human subjects research.* Chapel Hill, NC: University of North Carolina Press.

McLean, S., & Riley-Eddins, E. (2000). Recommended standards for culturally and linguistically appropriate health care services. *J Multicult Nurs Health, 6*(2), 5–6.

Pierce, C. (2001). The impact of culture on rural women's descriptions of health. *J Multicult Nurs Health, 7*(1), 50–53, 56.

Suzuki, L., Ponterottu, J. G., & Meller, P. J. (Eds.). (2001). *Handbook of multicultural assessment: Clinical, psychological, and educational applications.* San Francisco: Jossey-Bass.

Taylor, R. (2001). Multicultural communication: Are you culturally competent? *Nursing, 31*(4), 66.

Web Sites

Community and Family Health Administration (CHA and FHA), State of Maryland
http://mdpublichealth.org/

Community Health Assessments: Tools of the Trade (State of Pennsylvania)
http://www.hcwp.org/resources/commhealth/index.asp

Bureau of Primary Care, Department of Health and Human Services
http://bphc.hrsa.gov

Online Journal of Issues in Nursing: Multicultural Health Resources
http://www.library.kent.edu/~bschloma/hivaids/culture.htm

THE HOME VISIT

evaluation
home health care team
home visits
nursing process

primary intervention
standard precautions
telemedicine
termination

INTRODUCTION

Community health nurses often need to conduct home visits in the course of their practice. Many third-party payers encourage **home visits,** because it often costs less to provide care at home than in an institutional setting. This chapter discusses the advantages and disadvantages of the home visit as well as outlining practice guidelines.

KEY POINTS

1. The goals of community health nursing are often met through providing health care to families in their homes. Home health care visits can be provided by:

   A. visiting nurse associations
   B. hospice
   C. public health departments

   D. home health agencies
   E. school districts

2. Advantages of home visits:

   A. These visits cost less than hospital care, with better outcomes, espe-
       cially when chronic health issues are involved.
   B. Clients have greater control over their health and lives.
   C. The community health nurse gains access to families to provide health
       education and other prevention strategies.
   D. The nurse can observe family and environment factors that influence
       health.
   E. Home visits allow for **primary intervention,** to prevent disease or
       injury from occurring.
   F. Home visits facilitate family participation and promote family focus.

3. Disadvantages of home visits:

   A. The nurse's skills, personality, or physical ability may not be compati-
       ble with providing home visits.
   B. Home visits are time consuming; travel time is required to get to the
       persons needing care.
   C. There is no easy access to emergency equipment or consultation with
       other health professionals if needed.
   D. Home visits may present issues regarding the nurse's personal safety
       in some community or family settings.
   E. The nurse has less control over the care setting (for example, cleanli-
       ness, noise, privacy, or distractions).
   F. The family may resent the time the nursing visit requires, or they may
       begrudge the attention the client is receiving.
   G. Having a sick or needy family member in the home can result in care-
       giver exhaustion and illness.

4. Visit precautions for the nurse performing a home visit:

   A. Identify all exits.
   B. If someone in the home is using drugs or alcohol, do essential tasks for
       the client and leave.
   C. Any time you are concerned for your safety, leave immediately.
   D. Be aware of pets in the house and that they might perceive you as a
       threat. Ask the client or a family member to place a pet in another
       room if necessary.
   E. Do not attempt to intervene in domestic arguments.
   F. If the family offers something to eat or drink, politely refuse it,
       explaining that you are working. If offering food is a key part of the
       family's culture, ask if you can take the food with you.

    G. Follow your agency's policy for reporting threats, potentially harmful situations, and so forth.

5. The community health nurse develops objectives for primary, secondary, and tertiary prevention levels, in consultation with the family. To accomplish these objectives, the nurse needs to:

    A. assess client's ability or willingness to comply with treatment directions and/or change certain behaviors

    B. anticipate family needs, such as the timing of visits, the need to educate family members, respite care, and so on

6. When making a home visit, the community health nurse should use a fully equipped nursing bag.

    A. Requirements include equipment for basic assessment, medical asepsis, and waste disposal.

    B. **Standard precautions** to prevent the spread of pathogens must be observed. These precautions must be followed to avoid contamination from blood, body secretions, excretions, or contaminated items:

        i. wash hands (or use an alcohol-based handrub)
        ii. use gloves
        iii. wear eye and face protection
        iv. wear gown
        v. handle client care equipment carefully
        vi. clean environmental surfaces
        vii. use proper sharps disposal container

7. The community health nurse doing home visits usually works as part of a **home health care team** that can includes social workers, rehabilitation specialists, and home health nurses or aides. Cooperation and communication with other care providers are essential.

8. Implementing the **nursing process** in the home includes assessment, interviewing, observation, nursing diagnosis, and care planning. Nurses should also assess for cultural health practices to help understand client behavior and plan interventions more effectively.

9. The three most common interventions in home health care include:

    A. helping families deal with stress created by health problems

    B. making referrals for community services

    C. teaching and educating clients, with the focus on strengths rather than weaknesses

10. **Evaluation** is the ongoing process that continually assesses clients' progress toward expected outcomes.

11. **Termination** of home visits occurs when both client and nurse are satisfied that goals have been met or that appropriate referrals have been made.

12. An emerging trend is **telemedicine** and telecare, which use phone and computer technologies to monitor clients and provide care without the nurse making a home visit.

REVIEW ACTIVITIES

Questions

1. A client being treated for chronic emphysema would benefit from home visits because:
    a. care outcomes from home visits are better than hospitalization, especially for chronic conditions
    b. the community health nurse can bring in any needed equipment for the client
    c. the family is relieved of having to care for the client
    d. the nurse will not be distracted by family members or visitors

2. Which of the following identifies a disadvantage of home visits?
    a. There may not be a place for the nurse to wash his or her hands.
    b. It takes a lot of time and effort for the nurse to travel from client to client.
    c. Family members might try to take up the nurse's time with their own complaints.
    d. All of the above

3. To accomplish client care and prevention strategies, the nurse needs to:
    a. leave a brochure or booklet instructing the client what to do between visits
    b. keep the family from interfering with client treatment and education
    c. determine both the client's abilities to comply with treatment and the family's needs
    d. tell the family what to do but not bother the client, who is sick

4. Basic equipment needed for the nursing bag would include:
    a. stethoscope, antiseptic wipes, and sharps disposal box
    b. blood pressure cuff, tissues, and cell phone for emergencies

c. stethoscope, blood pressure cuff, and baggies

d. blood pressure cuff, narcotics, and sharps disposal box

5. The most effective way to implement the nursing process in the home would be:

a. using interview notes of the social worker to provide more efficient client care

b. assessing, interviewing, observing, making a nursing diagnosis, and planning care

c. having the client or family fill out a "multicultural assessment" questionnaire before beginning any assessment or interview, to avoid being culturally insensitive

d. conducting a client education session, making sure to focus on the client's strengths rather than weaknesses

6. Termination of home visits is appropriate when:

a. the client dies

b. the family requests it

c. care planning and assessment are complete

d. goals are met or appropriate referrals for other care made

Critical-Thinking Questions

1. Discuss the three most common interventions in home health care. How does each one of these help contribute to the health of the client?

2. A community health nurse is providing a home visit for two young Hispanic children with asthma. The nurse notices the odor of cigarette smoke in the room, and that several windows are open, letting in drafts of cold air. The grandmother, who is keeping the children, says that the apartment was "stuffy" and that "it's bad for children not to have fresh air." Implement the nursing process for this visit. Note one key point for each of the five nursing process steps. Are there any cultural factors present that might impact your findings or care planning?

3. A family of a client you visit offers you food and a cup of strong, black coffee. You politely refuse, explaining that you are working, but you do not like the smell of the food and you do not drink caffeine. For this family, offering food and coffee is a key part of being hospitable to guests. What are some ways to respect this family's gift without making yourself eat and drink what you do not want or like? What are some things you could say to this family that would validate their gesture?

Discussion Questions

1. What agencies in your community provide home visits? How do clients find out about them? How do health professionals know about them?

2. Think of two neighborhoods or communities near where you live or work. What safety issues or concerns would a nurse conducting a home visit need to be aware of? Would you feel safe working in these neighborhoods as a visiting nurse? Why or why not?

3. For what populations in your community would telemedicine or telecare be appropriate? For which populations would they not be appropriate?

References

Alexy, B., Benjamin-Coleman, R., & Brown, S. (2001). Home healthcare and client outcomes. *Home Healthcare Nurse, 19*(4), 233–239.

American Nurses Association. (1986). *Task force to develop standards of nursing practice for home health care.* Kansas City, MO: American Nurses Association.

Anthony, D. (2000). Current issues in nursing informatics. *Nurse Researcher, 8*(2), 18–28.

Booth, K., & Luker, K. (1999). *A practical handbook for community health nurses: Working with children and their families.* Oxford: Blackwell Science.

Conner, K. A. (1999). *Continuing to care: Older Americans and their families.* New York: Falmer Press.

Dalby, D. M., Sellors, J. W., Fraser, F. D., Fraser, C., et al. (2000). Effect of preventive home visits by a nurse on the outcomes of frail elderly people in a community:

A randomized controlled trial. *Canadian Medical Association Journal, 162*(4), 497–500. Available at http://www.cma.ca/cmaj/vol-162/issue-4/0497.htm

Humphrey, C. J. (1998). *Home care nursing handbook* (3rd ed.). Gaithersburg, MD: Aspen.

Larson, E. L., et al. (2001). How clean is the home environment? A tool to assess home hygiene. *Community Health Nursing, 18*(3), 139–150.

Macduff, C., West, B., & Harvey, S. (2001). Telemedicine in rural care, part 1: Developing and evaluating a nurse-led initiative. *Nurs Stand, 15*(32), 33–38.

Macduff, C., West, B., & Harvey, S. (2001). Telemedicine in rural care, part 2: Assessing the wider issues. *Nurs Stand, 15*(33), 33–37.

Meyers, D. (1997). *Client teaching guides for home health care.* Gaithersburg, MD: Aspen.

Pyne, R. H., & Pyne, R. (1998). *Professional discipline in nursing, midwifery, and health visiting.* Oxford: Blackwell Science.

Quinn, C. (2001). Analysis of the Home Health Symptom Management Model. *Lippincott Case Manage, 6*(3), 104–111.

Stackhouse, J. C. (1998). *Into the community: Nursing in ambulatory and home care.* Philadelphia: Lippincott.

Web Sites

American Telemedicine Association
http://www.atmeda.org/

Muskeg Lake Croe Nation
http://www.muskeglake.com/pshealthdiv.htm

National Association for Homecare and Hospice
http://www.nahc.org

Telemedicine Information Exchange (TIE)
http://www.tie.telemed.org/homehealth/

Visiting Nurse Association of America
http://www.vna.org

CHAPTER

8

ASSESSING FAMILIES

KEY TERMS

blended family

coping mechanisms

ecomap

extended family

family

family assessment

family health tree

family myths

family of origin

family of procreation

genogram

nuclear family

physical environment

primary prevention

pseudomutuality

psychological environment

scapegoating

secondary prevention

social environment

triangulation

INTRODUCTION

Working in a community setting generally involves working with families. Community health nurses must therefore understand the interactions and dynamics of families so that they can provide appropriate family assessment, planning, intervention, and evaluation. This chapter discusses the changing definitions of family, the characteristics of families, and the assessment of families.

KEY POINTS

1. The traditional definition of **family** is two or more persons related by birth, marriage, or adoption who reside together in a household. Today a broader concept or definition or family is used. This family is:

A. more inclusive
B. less structured
C. voluntary
D. not rule-bound
E. possibly time-limited

2. The following terms are often used to describe different family configurations:

   A. **nuclear family:** husband, wife, and their immediate children (biological or adopted, or both)
   B. **family of origin:** the family unit into which a person is born
   C. **family of procreation:** family created for the purpose of raising children
   D. **extended family:** the nuclear family plus other persons related by blood; this definition can also extend to voluntary, non-blood-related relationships
   E. **blended family:** a family made from two divorced families joined through remarriage

3. Families come in many forms and these alternate configurations are increasingly common. They can include:

   A. legally married: traditionally married, co-parenting, joint custody, and remarried
   B. dual-career: both adults in the family work outside the home
   C. foster families: provide a safe place for children separated from parent(s)
   D. childless by choice: adults in the family voluntarily decide not to have children
   E. never married: includes same-sex couples, single parents, and cohabitation
   F. multiadult household: includes multilateral marriage (three or more people in primary relationship with at least two other people in the group) and intentional communities
   G. extramarital: includes co-primary relationships (one or both members have a primary relationship with at least two partners, who may or may not know about each other) and open marriage
   H. extended: includes adult children living at home, parents, grandparents, or siblings

4. Characteristics associated with families include the following:

   A. affection, love, care, and compassion
   B. a sense of belonging and of history and place

C. family rituals for rejoicing and grieving
D. systems for earning money, supporting partners and children
E. sharing of labor, chores required to keep the family running

5. Family environment consists of physical, psychological, and social environments:

A. **physical environment**—which includes:
    i. housing and the conditions inside, outside, and surrounding it
    ii. any existing safety or environmental hazards
    iii. the amount and quality of services available

B. **psychological environment**—which includes:
    i. family dynamics
    ii. family strengths and weaknesses
    iii. communication skills
    iv. family roles
    v. family members' ability to cope with change or physical or psychological distress

C. **social environment**—which includes:
    i. religion
    ii. race or ethnicity
    iii. culture
    iv. socioeconomic class
    v. resources available such as through school, church, or community outlets

6. For the community health nurse, **family assessment** includes assessment of

A. how family members function with one another
B. how the family relates to the larger community

7. Community health nurses need to identify family strengths as well as weaknesses as part of a family assessment. These can include:

A. ability to recognize and meet other family members' needs
B. sensitivity to the needs or wishes of other family members
C. positive relations between family members
D. positive relations between the family and different parts of the community (church, school, neighborhood, etc.)
E. ability to grow from experiences and to maintain growth-enhancing relationships, whether between adults or between adults and children
F. ability to accept help from others

    G.   the ability to provide self-help when appropriate

    H.   flexibility of family roles

8. All families undergo stress. Different families have differing capacities for coping with stressful events.

9. Vulnerable families are those whose physical and emotional resources are insufficient to the point that functioning is threatened.

10. Vulnerable families have **coping mechanisms** that tend to be distorted or ineffective and that do not solve their problems. In fact, these mechanisms may further strain their meager resources.

11. Dysfunctional coping mechanisms include:

    A.   denying the problem exists

    B.   exploiting family members through abuse, neglect, or violence

    C.   **family myths:** for example,

        i.   "We're a happy family; no one is ever sad in our family."

        ii.   "Mom is fragile and needs to be protected. We won't tell her any bad news."

        iii.   These myths distort perceptions and stifle growth and adaptation.

    D.   **triangulation:** the strategy of drawing in a third person to absorb and reduce tension between two people

    E.   **scapegoating:** blaming someone instead of dealing with the issue

    F.   **pseudomutuality:** maintaining family status at the expense of family function

12. Family assessment tools that can be used include:

    A.   **genogram:** a graphic picture of family history, usually over three or more generations. The genogram maps such information as:

        i.   relationships among family members

        ii.   important life events

        iii.   places of residence

        iv.   characteristics such as race, culture, and religious affiliations

    B.   **family health tree:** a record of diseases that occur in a family. A family health tree can be used to track:

        i.   diseases that have genetic bases

        ii.   environmental diseases

        iii.   mental health disorders

C. **ecomap:** a picture of the family's patterns. Nurses can use an ecomap to identify:

   i. family resources that are present
   ii. family needs
   iii. conflicts
   iv. connections that are present or absent
   v. the balance or lack of balance between a family's needs and the resources available to the family

13. Two systems of nursing diagnosis:

A. NANDA system: uses nursing diagnostic labels
B. Omaha system: developed for community health nurses; consists of:

   i. problem classification
   ii. intervention
   iii. problem rating scale for outcomes

14. Planning and intervention for families must be in partnership with family members, not imposed from the outside by the community health nurse.

15. Primary prevention identifies actions to prevent occurrence of disease or dysfunction in families. It can include:

A. anticipatory guidance (teaching parents about upcoming developmental stages of children)
B. preparing for family changes (return to family of member who has been away, such as in hospital, prison, etc.)

16. Secondary prevention provides early recognition and treatment of existing health problems in families. It can include:

A. dealing with interactive factors that contribute to family dysfunction
B. emphasizing screening to detect problems before they become a burden or crisis for the family

17. Tertiary prevention treats existing diseases or conditions and focuses on preventing return of the problem. It can include:

A. helping a homeless family find permanent housing and connections to social services
B. providing care for a diabetic family member, and working to prevent diabetes-related complications through use of blood glucose monitoring, exercise, and diet

18. Evaluation begins with examining outcomes of care objectives. Each new piece of data requires new evaluation of the status of family care.

REVIEW ACTIVITIES

Questions

1. Which of the following statements about families is true?
   a. They are always made up of people who are related by birth or adoption.
   b. The current definition of family is much less flexible than it was in the past.
   c. Alternate family configurations are increasingly common.
   d. Never-married couples are not included under the definition of family.

2. A nuclear family of husband, wife, and immediate children plus other persons related by blood, or voluntary relationships is called a(n):
   a. blended family
   b. family of procreation
   c. family of origin
   d. extended family

3. An extramarital family configuration is characterized by:
   a. both adults in the family working outside the home
   b. child abuse
   c. open marriage or co-primary relationships
   d. adults who voluntarily decide not to have children

4. The family living in Anytown USA consists of two adults who are cohabiting and four children from previous relationships. The adults adhere to strict traditional gender roles and expect the children to be respectful and obedient to the adults in the household. This description tells about the family's:
   a. social environment
   b. psychological environment
   c. community environment
   d. dysfunction

5. A family's social environment consists of:
   a. family members' communication skills
   b. housing conditions inside and outside the house
   c. the extended family status
   d. religion, race, and socioeconomic class

6. Which of the following would be considered appropriate parts of a family assessment by a community health nurse?

   a. relationships between family members and between the family and community
   b. ability of family members to grow, help one another, and help themselves
   c. ability of family members to be flexible about roles and responsibilities
   d. all of the above

7. Which of the following would be considered a dysfunctional coping strategy?

   a. making a genogram
   b. triangulation
   c. role flexibility
   d. addressing the problem

8. A family that copes with a stressful situation by saying, "Our family is always upbeat, no matter what happens" is using which of the following dysfunctional coping strategies?

   a. pseudomutuality
   b. scapegoating
   c. triangulation
   d. family myth

9. A family health tree is used to track which of the following?

   a. mental health disorders that occur in a family
   b. marriage and divorce
   c. health conditions with no genetic basis
   d. places of residence

10. Which of the following is useful for showing the difference between a family's needs and the resources that are available to them?

   a. Omaha system
   b. family health tree
   c. ecomap
   d. genogram

Critical-Thinking Questions

1. The family in the apartment down the street is made up of four adults (two men, two women) ranging in age from 25 to 50, and six children (three girls, three boys), ranging in age from 3 months to 14 years. The

youngest adult woman is pregnant. Everyone in the family calls the oldest adult "mama," although she says she's never had any children. All of the adults seem very close and are physically affectionate, but they all say that they are not married. What are the possible family configurations that this group could fit? Why?

2. Describe and identify key components of family physical environment, psychological environment, and social environment. How do these environments act and interact to affect family function?

3. Describe a scenario that illustrates a family using:
   - triangulation
   - scapegoating
   - pseudomutuality

4. For the community health nurse, what are the advantages and disadvantages of using the NANDA nursing diagnosis system versus the Omaha system?

Discussion Questions

1. In your community, what is the most common family configuration? Has it changed significantly in the past five years? How?

2. How is your current family configuration similar to or different than the family configuration in which you grew up?

3. For a family with whom you have worked, list the key features of their physical, psychological, and social environment. How do these environments vary with different families in different parts of your community?

4. For families in your community, what are the advantages and disadvantages of using assessment tools such as the genogram, family health tree, or ecomap?

References

Barry, P. (2001). *Mental health and mental illness* (7th ed.). Philadelphia: Lippincott.

Chesla, C. A., & Rungreangkulkij, S. (2001). Nursing research on family processes in chronic illness in ethnically diverse families: A decade review. *J Fam Nursing,* 7(3), 230–243.

Craft-Rosenberg, M., Denehy, J. (Eds.). (2001). *Nursing interventions for infants, children, and families.* Thousand Oaks, CA: Sage.

Early, B. P., Smith, E. D., Todd, L., & Beem, T. (2000). The needs and supportive networks of the dying: An assessment instrument and mapping procedure for hospice patients. *Am J Hosp Palliat Care* 17(2):87–96.

Friedman, M. M. (1998). *Research* (4th ed.). Stamford, CT: Appleton & Lange.

Suzuki, L., Ponterorro, J., & Meller, P. J. (Eds.). (2001). *Handbook of multicultural assessment: Clinical, psychological, and educational applications.* San Francisco: Jossey-Bass.

Tagliareni, M. E., & Marckx, B. B. (1999). *Teaching in the community: Preparing nurses for the 21st century.* Sudbury, MA: Jones & Bartlett.

White, L. (2001). *Foundations of nursing: Caring for the whole person.* Clifton Park, NY: Delmar Learning.

Web Sites

Families, Systems, and Health: *Family Healthcare Journal*
http://www.fsh.org/

North American Nursing Diagnosis Association
http://www.nanda.org

Omaha System
http://www.omahasystem.org

U.S. Census Bureau: Families and Living Arrangements
http://www.census.gov/population/www/socdemo/hn-fam.html

U.S. Society and Values, "The American Family," Department of State, International Information Programs
http://usinfo.state.gov/journals/itsv/0101/ijse0101.htm

LEGAL ISSUES

breach of duty	living will
compensatory damages	malpractice
disciplinary action	medication errors
documentation error	negligence
durable power of attorney	Patient Self Determination Act
health care proxy	punitive damages

INTRODUCTION

Nurses operating in a community setting need to be aware of various legal considerations. This chapter reviews the broad legal environment that a community health nurse practices within and describes some steps that a nurse may take to reduce risk.

KEY POINTS

1. *Bleiler v. Bodnar* established a case law standard for nursing malpractice. Previously, nurses could only commit negligence, not malpractice.

2. Elements of professional **negligence** (**malpractice**) are as follows:

A. Duty

    i. Duty hinges on the professional relationship between the nurse and the client.

    ii. When a client enters a facility's or agency's care, duty is automatically established.

B. **Breach of duty**

    i. Nurses are required to act as any reasonably prudent nurse would act.

    ii. Breach occurs if the nurse does not do something that should have been done, or does something that should not have been done.

    iii. Nurses must meet acceptable standards of care:

        a. internal standards set by agency: policies and procedures, job description

        b. external standards: Nurse Practice Act of state where practicing, American Nurses Association

        c. other legal regulations or professional standards of practice

        d. published standards: literature, specialty organizations

        e. formal and continuing education

        f. expert testimony and case law

C. The nurse can commit breach of duty in the following ways:

    i. medication errors

    ii. failure to use sterile technique

    iii. failure to notify physician in a timely manner

    iv. failure to follow physician orders or following inappropriate orders

    v. improper monitoring or assessment

    vi. improper use of equipment

    vii. failure to follow appropriate protocol

    viii. failure to provide proper client care

D. An agency or facility can commit breach of duty by the following:

    i. insufficient equipment

    ii. insufficient equipment maintenance

    iii. insufficient staffing

E. Causation

    i. determination of whether the nurse's conduct was directly responsible for the injury to the client

    ii. legal standard is "caused or contributed to cause"

    iii. client's actions can also contribute to the cause of injury (for example, if the client did not follow the plan of care)

F. Damages/Injury

    i. usually classified as physical injury but can include emotional distress

    ii. may be classified as **compensatory damages,** for economic (lost wages, etc.) or noneconomic (pain and suffering) losses

    iii. may be classified as **punitive damages,** to punish the wrongdoer, especially if the nurse's action was seen as in total disregard for the client's well-being

    iv. falsifying medical records can trigger punitive damages

3. Licensure and disciplinary matters also affect nurses. Each state has its own practice act and disciplinary process.

4. The board of nursing for each state establishes:

A. rule making
B. licensing authority
C. authority to conduct and participate in cases involving nurses licensed in that state
D. administration and enforcement of the Nurse Practice Act

5. According to the American Nurses Association (1986), the grounds for disciplinary action against nurses include:

A. violation of the Nurse Practice Act
B. addiction to or dependence on alcohol or other drugs
C. habitual use of narcotics
D. falsifying client records, or failure to record
E. unprofessional conduct that is likely to deceive, defraud, or harm the public
F. being convicted of a felony or crime involving moral turpitude
G. negligent or willful violation of nursing practice standards
H. committing unlawful acts such as practicing nursing without a license or using a fraudulent license
I. helping others obtain fraudulent licensing or credentials

6. The eight categories of **disciplinary action** under which a nurse's actions can be classified are:

A. fraud and deceit
B. criminal activity
C. negligence, risk to clients, physical or mental incapacity (unsafe practitioners)
D. violation of Nurse Practice Act or rules

E. disciplinary action by another jurisdiction
F. incompetence
G. unethical conduct
H. drug and alcohol use

7. The actions that a state nursing board can take against a nurse include:

A. denying application for licensure
B. suspending current license or placing the nurse on probation
C. revoking license
D. requiring the nurse to submit to "care, counseling, or treatment" to get or maintain license
E. administering a public or private reprimand
F. reinstating license

8. Risk management strategies include preventing the incidents that most often lead to malpractice claims: deficiencies in the medical record, adverse outcomes, and complications

9. Be sure to follow your agency's policy for documentation. Key points to avoid **documentation error** include the following:

A. Make sure everything written is legible and easily understood.
B. Record objectively, thoroughly, and carefully, making sure to cite facts, not opinions.
C. Avoid documenting anything you did not see or cannot verify.

10. Good documentation techniques are particularly important for the community health care setting.

11. Another key area is to reduce the risk of **medication errors.** Nurses should:

A. help community members learn about medications taken for acute and chronic illnesses, drug interactions, and resources in the community for information about medications

12. The **Patient Self Determination Act** became effective in October 1991. The law requires hospitals, nursing facilities, providers of home care or personal care services, hospice programs, and health maintenance organizations that receive Medicare and Medicaid funding to have policies about advanced directives such as:

A. **living will:** precise treatment wishes under certain conditions, such as a debilitating illness, Alzheimer's disease, and the like.

B. **durable power of attorney:** names a decision maker in case the client loses the ability to make his or her own treatment decisions. Also called a **health care proxy.**

13. Organizations and agenices can face legal action if they fail to comply with the requirements of the Patient Self-Determination Act.

REVIEW ACTIVITIES

Questions

1. Which of the following is a true statement about nursing legal issues?
   a. Nurses can be charged with negligence but not malpractice.
   b. A clear legal standard does not exist for nursing malpractice.
   c. Nurses employed by an agency are assumed to have an automatic duty to clients of the facility and are assigned to them.
   d. None of the above

2. Which of the following standards can set standards of care for nurses?
   a. published standards such as professional literature
   b. state and national Nurse Practice Acts
   c. case law
   d. all of the above

3. Which of the following would be considered a breach of duty?
   a. notifying a physician promptly of a client's reaction to a medication
   b. checking the skin reaction 48 hours after administering a PPD
   c. following physician orders to give Amoxicillin to a client who is allergic to penicillin in a public health clinic
   d. changing gloves between checking a client's blood glucose and removing a dressing from a venous leg ulcer

4. Punitive damages are awarded to:
   a. compensate a client for lost wages plus pain and suffering
   b. help the client pay for the expenses associated with an illness or injury
   c. avoid sending a nurse to court for malpractice
   d. punish the person who committed the wrong

5. A nurse in any state can incur formal disciplinary action from the state board of nursing for which of the following?
   a. habitual lateness and poor work ethic

    b.   off-duty drug and alcohol use, addiction, or dependence

    c.   conviction for a class I misdemeanor, excluding traffic tickets

    d.   habitual disrespect for a supervisor

6. A nursing board could institute which of the following disciplinary actions against a nurse?

    a.   suspending or revoking a nurse's license

    b.   levying a fine equal to 10 percent of the nurse's current salary

    c.   filing suit against a nurse in court for malpractice and related damages

    d.   refusing to allow a nurse to get counseling for alcohol or drug abuse while licensed

7. Which of the following statements is true?

    a.   Agencies that receive Medicare and Medicaid funding are not required to comply with the Patient Self Determination Act.

    b.   The Patient Self Determination Act determines reasons for filing malpractice suits if it finds causation of injury to a client.

    c.   Living wills are applicable only if the hospital or agency finds the client's choice morally acceptable.

    d.   A health care proxy only names the decision maker; it does not specify the decision.

Critical-Thinking Questions

1. A nurse in a public health clinic inadvertently writes the incorrect dosage of a medication on a client's chart. When doing a chart review at the end of shift, the nurse notices the discrepancy, corrects it by using whiteout to cover the mistake, and then writes the correct medication dosage over the old figure. Could this nurse be a candidate for disciplinary action? If so, which one? If not, why not?

2. You visit a 70-year-old woman who is being treated for advanced congestive heart failure. She says she does not want any more treatment, that she is tired and just wants to be comfortable so she can die in peace. You check her records. There is a health care proxy naming her son as her decision maker. Her files do not indicate a living will. A few minutes after her son arrives at her home to visit, the client loses consciousness. Her son says, "Do everything you can to save her—a heart transplant if you have to." What do you do?

Discussion Questions

1. Have you read the Nurse Practice Act for your state? Where can you find it? Is it different from those of neighboring states? In what way?

2. Of the eight categories of disciplinary action, which one is adjudicated most often in your state?

References

Beckmann, J. P. (2000). *Nursing malpractice: Implications for clinical practice and nursing education.* New York: Galen Press.

Carruth, A. K., & Booth, D. (1999). Disciplinary actions against nurses: Who is at risk? *J Nurs Law, 6*(3), 55–62.

Caulfield, H. (2001). Negligence. *Pract Nurse, 22*(5), 16, 18, 21.

Cowley, S., & Andrews, A. (2001). A scenario-based analysis of health visiting dilemmas. *Community Pract, 74*(4), 139–142.

Dupree, C. Y. (2000). The attitudes of black Americans toward advance directives. *J Transcult Nurs, 11*(1), 12–18.

Exstrom, S. M. (2001). The state board of nursing and its role in continued competency. *J Contin Educ Nurs, 32*(3), 118–125.

Frank-Stromborg, M., Christensen, A., & Do, D. (2001). Nurse documentation not done or worse, done the wrong way. *Oncol Nurs Forum, 28*(4), 697–702.

Gibson, T. (2001). Nurses and medication errors: A discursive reading of the literature. *Nurs Inquiry, 8*(2), 108–117.

Iyer, P. (2001). *Nursing malpractice* (2nd ed.). Tucson, AZ: Lawyers and Judges Publishing.

Milton, C. L. (2001). Ethical issues. Advance directives: living with certainty-uncertainty—a nursing perspective. *Nurs Sci Q, 14*(3), 195–198.

O'Keefe, M. E. (Ed.).(2000). Nursing practice and the law: Avoiding malpractice and other legal risks. Philadelphia: F. A. Davis.

Robinson, E. M. (2001). Ethical issues: Caring for incompetent patients and their surrogates: A case study of end-of-life care. *Am J Nurs, 101*(7), 75–76.

Scott, R. (1998). *Health care malpractice: A primer for legal issues for professionals* (2nd ed.). New York: McGraw-Hill.

Snider, M. J., & Hood, K. M. (2001). Legal and ethical issues: Confidentiality: Keeping secrets. *J Prof Nurs, 17*(5), 214–214.

Tammelleo, A. D. (2000). Legally speaking: Protecting patients' end-of-life choices. *RN, 63*(8), 75, 77, 79.

Ulrich, L. (2001). *The Patient Self-Determination Act: Meeting the challenges in patient care.* Washington, DC: Georgetown University Press.

Web Sites

National Council of State Boards of Nursing
http://www.ncsbn.org

Nursing Protection Group
http://www.npg.com/index.php

Nursing Center Professional Development Legal/Ethical
http://www.nursingcenter.com/prodeu/ce_list.asp?flag=cdt&id=229824

Patient Self Determination Act: Final Regulations
http://www.dgcenter.org/acp/pdf/pdsa.pdf

Position Statements on Nursing and the Patient Self Determination Act
http://nursingworld.org/readroom/position/ethics/etsdet.htm

Part III

What Populations Do Community Health Nurses Serve?

SELECTED COMMUNICABLE DISEASES

agent
communicable disease
E. coli
Ebola
endemic
epidemic
hantavirus
hepatitis
host

infectious disease
influenza
Lyme disease
multidrug-resistant tuberculosis
pandemic
pediculosis
rabies
scabies
tuberculosis

INTRODUCTION

A key role of the community health nurse is the prevention and treatment of communicable diseases. This chapter describes the language of communicable disease and discusses the goals nurses use in evaluating the success of disease prevention programs. It also examines common communicable diseases that community health nurses are likely to encounter in their practices.

KEY POINTS

1. Key concepts for communicable diseases:

    A. **communicable disease:** A disease or illness in a susceptible host, caused by a potentially harmful infectious organism or its toxic byproducts. Communicable disease spreads due to contact between an infectious agent and a susceptible host.

B. **infectious disease:** A disease or illness caused by an infectious agent entering the body of a susceptible host and then developing or growing.

C. **host:** A person or other living being that can be infected by an organism.

D. **infectious agent:** An organism that causes infectious disease. Agents can be:

    i. bacteria
    ii. fungi
    iii. viruses
    iv. metazoa
    v. protozoa

E. **agent:** Something that must be present in the environment for a disease to occur in a susceptible host.

F. **endemic:** When an infectious agent or disease has a constant presence within a defined geographic area.

G. **epidemic:** Occurrences of an infectious agent or disease that clearly exceed the usual expected frequency of the disease in a particular population—for example, an influenza epidemic, when a large number of elderly people in a city get the flu.

H. **pandemic:** When an epidemic outbreak occurs worldwide (such as HIV infection).

2. Healthy People 2010 objectives for communicable disease:

A. increase the number of local health departments with culturally appropriate and linguistically competent community health promotion and disease prevention programs

B. reduce the occurrence of vaccine-preventable diseases, through education, outreach, and access to vaccinations

C. target diseases that are significant in certain populations, such as HIV; hepatitis A, B, C; bacterial meningitis; and tuberculosis

3. **Multidrug-resistant tuberculosis.** Bacterial infection of the lungs.

A. Symptoms include

    i. fever
    ii. cough
    iii. expectorating blood (hemoptysis)
    iv. chest pain
    v. weight loss

B. Some TB bacteria have become drug-resistant.

C. Vulnerable populations include:

      i. poor, homeless people without access to health care or follow-up

     ii. immigrants from countries where TB is endemic

   iii. people with HIV infection and compromised immune systems

   iv. anyone with poor access to health care for follow-up

D. Primary prevention: educating the public about the need to complete the entire course of drug treatment

E. Secondary prevention: minimizing the disease's ability to spread throughout the community; preventing treatment failures from individuals with poor compliance with the lengthy, potentially complicated therapy program

F. Treatment: multidrug regimem with direct observation therapy to ensure compliance

4. Tuberculosis

A. Vulnerable populations: children, persons with HIV infection, persons in congregate living such as prisons, shelters, long-term care facilities, and dormitories

B. Primary prevention strategies include:

      i. health promotion and education

     ii. skin testing (PPD)

   iii. education on behaviors to reduce risk of transmission from infected persons

   iv. education about environmental factors (sunlight, ventilation) that can reduce transmission

C. Secondary prevention strategies include:

      i. screening high-risk populations

     ii. early diagnosis and treatment

D. Tertiary prevention strategies include:

      i. monitoring long-term health status

     ii. direct observation of therapy to ensure compliance with treatment

E. Community health nurses have a key role in tuberculosis prevention and treatment. They can

      i. identify people at risk

     ii. initiate testing programs

   iii. do follow-up for compliance

   iv. provide education

5. *E. coli:* 01557:H7. This bacteria (0157:H7 is one of hundreds of strains) is spread through contaminated food.

A. Some infected people have no symptoms; others develop bloody diarrhea and abdominal cramps.
B. In some cases *E. coli* infection can lead to kidney failure.
C. Vulnerable populations: children, adults with compromised immune systems
D. Prevention: radiation of beef before it enters public food supply; adequate handwashing and proper cooking
E. Treatment: depends on the symptoms

6. **Lyme disease.** The Lyme disease bacterium (*Borrelia burgdorferi*) is transmitted when an infected deer tick bites a person.

A. A bull's-eye rash may appear at the site of the tick bite.
B. Early symptoms include flu-like aches and fatigue.
C. Later symptoms include severe fatigue, arthritis, and neurological and cardiac symptoms.
D. Vulnerable populations: people living in areas with infected ticks
E. Primary prevention strategies include:

  i. education about the disease
  ii. avoiding tick-endemic areas
  iii. inspecting for ticks
  iv. using insecticide and wearing proper light-colored clothing outdoors.

F. Secondary prevention strategies include:

  i. procedures for properly removing ticks
  ii. follow-up testing
  iii. early diagnosis before debilitating symptoms occur

G. Treatment: antibiotics. The sooner antibiotic therapy is started, after infection is confirmed, the better the results.

7. **Ebola.** Caused by a virus that can be spread from person to person, or through direct contact with infected blood, semen, or secretions.

A. Symptoms include bleeding in the mucosa, abdomen, pericardium, and vagina.
B. Death follows bleeding, shock, and respiratory failure.
C. Vulnerable populations:

  i. persons living in an area of outbreak
  ii. those exposed to persons with nosocomial infections
  iii. laboratory workers

D. Primary prevention strategy: Interrupting of the spread of the virus from person to person.

E. Secondary prevention strategy: Testing for the Ebola antibody.

F. Treatment: There is no cure for Ebola; mortality rate is around 90 percent.

8. **Hantavirus.** Respiratory disease caused by a virus that is carried and spread by rodents. Person-to-person transmission may also be possible.

A. Symptoms include:

    i. fever

    ii. interstitial edema

    iii. severe shortness of breath

    iv. joint pain, nausea, and vomiting (sometimes)

B. Vulnerable populations:

    i. people exposed to rodent feces and urine or contaminated materials

    ii. people bitten by rodents

C. Primary prevention strategies:

    i. rodent control in endemic areas

    ii. precautions for decontaminating suspected infectious areas

    iii. using protective clothing

D. Secondary prevention strategy: testing for hantavirus antibodies

E. Treatment: There is no cure, and mortality rate is about 45 percent. Supportive care such as controlling fever, providing respiratory support, or controlling hemorrhage is provided.

9. **Hepatitis.** An inflammation of the liver due to a number of possible causes, including bacteria, viruses, parasites, alcohol, drugs, or chemical toxins. There are different types of hepatitis but most display the same symptoms: jaundice, fever, nausea and vomiting, clay-colored stools, and dark urine.

A. Hepatitis A

    i. Vulnerable populations: persons exposed to unsanitary conditions, poor hygiene; those having sexual contact with infected persons; persons exposed to contaminated water or food such as shellfish

    ii. Prevention: Hepatitis A vaccine for those at risk for exposure

B. Hepatitis B

    i. Vulnerable populations: persons who have contact with blood or body fluid of infected person; persons who have sex with infected persons; people who share needles; newborns infected during birth

      ii. Primary prevention strategy: vaccination/immunization of children and at-risk adults (including health care workers)

     iii. Secondary prevention strategies: screening of high-risk populations, early detection

     iv. Tertiary prevention strategy: minimizing effects of the disease, especially liver damage

C. Hepatitis C

      i. Vulnerable populations: intravenous drug users and hemophiliacs receiving frequent blood transfusions; people who have sex with infected persons; people who have received blood and/or solid organs before 1992 (Centers for Disease Control and Prevention [CDC])

     ii. Primary and secondary prevention strategies: education and screening

    iii. Tertiary prevention strategies: assisting clients with chronic nature of disease, helping them find resources

D. Hepatitis D (Delta virus)

      i. Vulnerable populations: same as for hepatitis B

     ii. Prevention: vaccination

E. Hepatitis E (enteric non-A hepatitis)

      i. usually spread through contaminated water or by fecal-oral contamination

     ii. there is no diagnostic test available

    iii. has a 10 percent mortality rate in pregnant women

    iv. not common in the United States

10. Pediculosis. An infestation of lice, tiny insects that feed on human blood.

A. Head lice are usually spread by sharing combs and hats.

B. Pubic lice are usually spread through sexual contact with an infested person.

C. Body lice are spread through infested clothing and bed linens.

D. Main symptom is itching in the affected area.

E. Vulnerable populations:

      i. children (head lice)

     ii. sexually active people (pubic lice)

    iii. people with poor hygiene (body lice)

F. Prevention: screening; teaching children not to share combs, brushes, or caps

G. Treatment: removal of lice through specially formulated shampoos; removal of nits (eggs); washing clothing and bedding in very hot water and drying at highest temperature setting; discarding combs, brushes, and hair care items and replacing with new items when the eggs are all gone

   H. Note that treatment trends are currently moving away from the use of harsh insecticides due to their possible adverse effects on children.

11. Scabies. A skin disease caused by a tiny parasite (mite) that burrows under the skin.

   A. Characteristic welts are usually found:

      i. between the fingers
     ii. on the inside of the wrists
    iii. on the buttocks
    iv. in the axillae
     v. along the beltline

   B. Main symptom is intense itching, especially at night.
   C. Vulnerable populations: anyone who has contact with an infected person
   D. Prevention: education, avoiding direct contact with infected person; washing clothes or bed linens to prevent spread to other people
   E. Treatment: Insecticide lotions for killing mites

12. Influenza. Viral illness characterized by severe muscle aches, fever, headache, sore throat, and cough.

   A. Severe complications and death can accompany infection.
   B. Vulnerable populations: elderly people and those with chronic illnesses or compromised immune symptoms are more likely to develop severe complications.
   C. Primary prevention strategy: yearly vaccination for vulnerable populations and people who work with vulnerable populations and can be carriers
   D. Secondary prevention strategies:

      i. early diagnosis
     ii. identification of vulnerable populations
    iii. early treatment to prevent complications

13. Rabies. Viral illness occurring in mammals that may be spread to humans through contact with an infected animal.

   A. Early symptoms include:

      i. fever
     ii. headache

       iii. malaise

       iv. itching or numbness at the wound site

  B. Later symptoms include:

       i. difficulty swallowing

       ii. paralysis

       iii. agitation and disorientation, followed by coma and death

  C. Vulnerable populations: people at increased risk of contact with animals that carry rabies, especially raccoons, skunks, coyotes, foxes, and bats; or people with pets that are not vaccinated against rabies (these pets come in contact with infected animals, and then have contact with people)

  D. Primary prevention strategies: educating people about:

       i. vaccination of pets

       ii. animal control

       iii. avoiding wild animals, especially those that act oddly or look sick

       iv. not feeding wild animals

       v. preexposure vaccination for people whose work puts them at higher risk of contact with animals that carry rabies

14. Communicable diseases and the community health nurse's role

  A. Community health nurses often have the first contact with people with communicable diseases.

  B. Informed nurses can be instrumental in preventing disease spread using primary, secondary, and tertiary prevention methods.

REVIEW ACTIVITIES

Questions

1. An illness that spreads because of contact between an infectious agent and a susceptible host is called:

  a. endemic

  b. pandemic

  c. infectious agent

  d. communicable disease

2. The difference between endemic and epidemic is that:

    a.   endemic affects only elderly people while epidemic does not

    b.   epidemic affects a particular population while endemic affects a geographic area

    c.   endemic affects a particular population while epidemic affects a geographic area

    d.   endemic and epidemic, like pandemic, are worldwide in scope

3. The virus that causes an influenza epidemic would be classified as:

    a.   infectious disease

    b.   infectious agent

    c.   pandemic

    d.   target disease

4. Which of the following objectives for communicable disease are part of the Healthy People 2010 objectives?

    a.   increase the number of local health departments with staff that is multicultural or multilingual

    b.   reduce the number of people who get influenza

    c.   work to identify and treat drug-resistant tuberculosis in homeless populations

    d.   all of the above

5. Which of the following is true about multidrug-resistant tuberculosis?

    a.   It seldom occurs in immigrant populations.

    b.   Educating people about the need to complete drug treatment is a tertiary prevention strategy.

    c.   Treatment includes a five-drug regimen and does not require follow-up.

    d.   None of the above

6. Primary prevention strategies for tuberculosis include all of the following except:

    a.   immunization

    b.   skin testing

    c.   health promotion

    d.   education

7. An example of educating people to prevent *E. coli* infection would include:

    a.   urging people not to eat any hamburger to avoid infection

    b.   providing antibiotics for the diarrhea associated with *E. coli*

    c.   telling people how *E. coli* leads to kidney failure

    d.   showing people how to cook hamburger to the proper temperature

8. Which of the following is true about prevention strategies for Lyme disease?

   a.   If a bull's-eye rash appears, the disease cannot be prevented.
   b.   Early use of antibiotics once infection is confirmed produces better results.
   c.   Wearing proper clothing in tick-infested areas has little preventive value.
   d.   All of the above

9. A population that is exposed to rodent droppings or urine could be at risk for:

   a.   Ebola virus
   b.   hepatitis A
   c.   scabies
   d.   hantavirus

10. Which of the following is true about the Ebola virus?

   a.   It occurs only in Africa and Asia, not in the United States.
   b.   It cannot be spread from person to person.
   c.   The mortality rate is around 90 percent.
   d.   Blood tests in exposed people show no antibodies.

11. A community health nurse working in a town that has an outbreak of hantavirus could perform which of the following primary prevention measures?

   a.   Check community members for hantavirus antibodies in their blood.
   b.   Teach people how to control rodents and safely get rid of rodent droppings.
   c.   Distribute antibiotics to community members to prevent infection.
   d.   All of the above

12. Which of the following is commonly spread through sexual contact?

   a.   hepatitis B
   b.   hantavirus
   c.   rabies
   d.   none of the above

13. Which types of hepatitis can be prevented by vaccination?

   a.   All types of hepatitis can be prevented by vaccination.
   b.   No types of hepatitis can be prevented by vaccination.
   c.   All types except hepatitis C and E can be prevented by vaccination.
   d.   Only hepatitis A can be prevented by vaccination.

14. Which types of hepatitis are commonly contracted through contaminated food or water?

   a.   hepatitis A and E
   b.   hepatitis B and C
   c.   hepatitis A and C
   d.   hepatitis D and E

15. The most effective treatment of pediculosis is:

    a. scratching the affected area

    b. removing lice and nits from body, clothes, and bedding

    c. immunization

    d. avoiding sharing hats and combs

16. The most effective primary strategy for preventing influenza in the residents of an assisted living facility would be:

    a. to immunize residents and staff against influenza

    b. to screen staff for influenza symptoms as they come to work

    c. to provide antibiotics to all residents beginning in November

    d. to hospitalize any residents who develop fever, body aches, or sore throat

17. An effective strategy to prevent elementary school children from contracting rabies would be to:

    a. give all children the rabies vaccine

    b. teach them never to approach or touch unknown or strange-acting animals

    c. examine the children to see if they have difficulty swallowing

    d. show the children how to properly feed wild animals

Critical-Thinking Questions

1. Identify the agent for the following:

- diaper rash
- influenza
- diarrhea
- heart disease
- chicken pox
- bronchitis

Which of these agents would be considered infectious?

2. Within the past 200 years, which epidemics can you think of that have become pandemic? Which diseases continue to be pandemic?

3. A community health nurse performs a home visit and checkup for a new mother and her baby. Lab tests for the mother come back positive for hepatitis B. What should the nurse's next steps be?

4. A community health nurse is speaking to students and teachers at an elementary school after an outbreak of head lice at a nearby school. What are the key teaching points that the nurse needs to make?

Discussion Questions

1. What agents or diseases are endemic to your community?

2. Has your community experienced an epidemic within the past year? Five years? What was it?

3. Choose a population in your community or area. Which diseases occur most often in this population? Are any of the diseases preventable through vaccination?

4. How well does your community meet the objectives for Healthy People 2010?

5. For the following populations in your community, what infectious/communicable diseases are they at risk for?
   - immigrants
   - IV drug users
   - children
   - sexually active people

6. In your community, how does the media portray incidences of communicable diseases (for example, infectious hepatitis, influenza, pediculosis, or tuberculosis)? If you feel that the media coverage is less than adequate, how could a community health nurse help improve it?

REFERENCES

Alan, B., and Bakalar, B. (2000). *Hepatitis A to G.* E-book. Digital download available from www.amazon.com.

Bartlett, J. (2001). *2001–2002 pocket book of infectious disease therapy* (11th ed.). Philadelphia: Lippincott, Williams & Wilkins.

Campbell, G. D., & Payne, D. K. (Eds.). (2001). *Bone's atlas of pulmonary and critical care medicine* (2nd ed.). Philadelphia: Lippincott, Williams & Wilkins.

Capps, P. A., Pinger, R. R., Russell, K. M., & Wood, M. L. (1999). Community health nurses' knowledge of Lyme disease and implications for surveillance and community education. *J Community Health Nurs, 16*(1), 1–15.

Cerrato, P. (1999). When food is the culprit. *RN, 62*(6), 52–58,

Connolly, C. (2000). The TB preventorium: Tuberculosis. *Am J Nurs, 100*(10), 62–65, 91–92.

Connolly-Taylor, B. (2000). Controversies in the treatment and management of Lyme disease. *J Intravenous Nurs, 23*(1), 15–20.

Day, M. W. (2001). Action stat: E. coli food poisoning. *Nursing, 31*(6), 96.

Galin, J. I., Fauci, A., Liang, T., Hofnagle, J. (Eds.). (2000). *Hepatitis C (A volume in the biomedical research reports).* San Diego: Academic Press.

Ghani, S. (2001). Convincing an Asian community of the importance of flu vaccination. *Prof Nurse, 17*(2), 130.

Hensel, P. (2000). The challenge of choosing a pediculicide. *Public Health Nurs, 17*(4), 300–304.

Higson, E. (2001). Flu in the community: Nursing management. *Nurs Times, 97*(5), 35–36.

Hitchcock, J., Schubert, P., & Thomas, S. (1999). *Community health nursing: Caring in action.* Clifton Park, NY: Delmar Learning.

Ibarra, J. (2001). Head lice: Changing the costly chemotherapy culture. *J Community Nurs, 6*(3), 146, 148–151.

Jossi, K. (2001). Lyme disease: An in-depth look at a formidable infection. *J Emerg Nurs, 101*(9), 461–470.

Larson, E., & Duarte, C. G. (2001). Home hygiene practices and infectious disease symptoms among household members. *Public Health Nurs, 18*(2), 116–127.

Niederman, M. S., Savosi, G. A., & Glassroth, J. (Eds.). (2000). *Respiratory infections* (2nd ed.). Philadelphia: Lippincott, Williams & Wilkins.

Palmer, S., and Parry, S. (2002). *E. coli: Environmental health issues of VTEC 0157.* Routledge.

Parini, S. (2001). Infection control special report: Hepatitis: speaking out about the silent epidemic. *Nurs Manage, 32*(6), 18–24.

Porter-Jones, G. (2001). Developing local TB guidelines. *Nurs Times, 97*(26), 59.

Reichman, L. B., & Hershfeld, E. S. (Eds.). (2000). *Tuberculosis: A comprehensive international approach.* Marcel Dekker.

Ryan, K. (Ed.). (1994). *Sherris medical microbiology: An introduction to infectious diseases.* Norwalk, CT: Appleton & Lange.

Smith, L. S. (2001). Health of America's newcomers. *Community Health Nurs, 18*(1), 53–68.

Stanhope, M. (1997). *Public and community health nurses consultant: A health promotion guide.* St. Louis, MO: Mosby.

Strydom, M., Greeff, M., & Nel, A. (2000). Guidelines for implementation in the education-learning situation regarding tuberculosis. *Curationis, 23*(4), 82–89.

Venna, S., Flesicher, A. B. Jr., & Feldman, S. R. (2001). Scabies and lice: Review of the clinical features and management principles. *Dermatol Nurs, 13*(4), 257–262, 265–266.

Wade, C. F. (2000). Keeping Lyme disease at bay: An integrated approach to prevention. *Am J Nurs, 100*(7), 26–32.

Walker, L. (2001). Ebola haemorrhagic fever. *Nurs Stand, 15*(32), 40–42.

Washer, P. (2001). Hepatitis C: Transmission, treatment and occupational risk. *Nurs Stand, 15*(40), 43–46.

White, L. (2001). *Foundations of nursing: Caring for the whole person.* Clifton Park, NY: Delmar Learning.

Willock, K. M., Goodrow, B., & Meyers, P. L. (2000). News, notes & tips: Community-based mock epidemic. *Nurse Educ, 25*(1), 42, 47.

Web Sites

American Lyme Disease Foundation
http://www.aldf.com/

Association for Professionals in Infection Control and Epidemiology
http://www.apic.org/

Centers for Disease Control and Prevention
http://www.cdc.gov/ (search for infectious diseases)

Department of Health and Human Services. Healthy People 2010
http://www.health.gov.healthypeople/

Emerging Infectious Disease Journal (CDC)
http://www.cdc.gov/ncidod/eid/

Federation of American Scientists (FAS) Program for Monitoring Emerging Diseases
http://www.fas.org/promed

Frequently asked questions about tuberculosis: World Health Organization
http://www.who.int/gov/nchstp/tb/faqs/qa.htm

Hepatitis B Foundation
http://www.hepb.org/

Hepatitis Foundation International
http://www.hepfi.org/

Hepatitis Home Page
http://www.cdc.gov/ncidod/diseases/hepatitis/

Hepatitis Information Network
http://www.hepnet.com

Hospital Infection Control Practices Advisory Committee (HICPAC)
http://www.cdc.gov/ncidod/hip/HICPAC/Hicpac.htm

International Conference on Emerging Infectious Diseases
http://www.asmusa.org/

Lyme Disease Foundation
http://www.lyme.org/

Lyme Disease Home Page
http://www.cdc.gov/ncidod/dvbid/lyme/

Medline Plus: E. coli infections
http://www.nlm.nih.gov/medlineplus/ecoliinfections.html

National Foundation for Infectious Diseases
http://www.nfid.org

National Pediculosis Association
http://www.headlice.org/doit4thekids/

Tuberculosis Network
http://www.tuberculosis.net

World Health Organization (WHO)
http://www.who.int/home-page/

World Wide Web Virtual Library: E. coli index
http://web.bham.ac.uk/bcm4ght6/res.html

CHAPTER 1

SEXUALLY TRANSMITTED DISEASES (STDs)

KEY TERMS

acquired immunodeficiency
   syndrome (AIDS)
carrier
chlamydia
cultural attitudes
gonorrhea
herpes simplex virus 2
human immunodeficiency virus
   (HIV)

human papillomavirus
primary prevention
secondary prevention
sexually transmitted diseases (STDs)
syphilis
tertiary prevention
trichomoniasis

INTRODUCTION

Although there are many types of communicable diseases, a major focus of a community health nurse's prevention efforts are sexually transmitted diseases (STDs), which are spread through sexual contact. This chapter will review the different types of STDs, their characteristics, and the role of the community health nurse in preventing the spread of STDs.

KEY POINTS

1. There are various types of communicable diseases. A major category is **sexually transmitted diseases** (STDs), which are spread through sexual contact.

A. STDs make up five of the 10 most frequently reported diseases in the United States.
B. Consequences of STDs range from mild symptoms, to serious or disabling illness, to death.
C. Barriers to the prevention and control of STDs include:

   i. societal and cultural factors, including reluctance to discuss sexuality or sexual habits and behaviors
   ii. behavioral and social stereotypes, such as double standards of sexual behavior for men and women
   iii. confusing or mixed media messages, such as simultaneously urging abstinence while using sexually explicit images in advertising

D. Dialogue about STDs is needed to facilitate primary prevention and risk reduction.
E. Populations at greatest risk for STD infection are:

   i. teens and young adults
   ii. women
   iii. intravenous drug users
   iv. African Americans
   v. Hispanics

F. Environmental factors that contribute to the spread of STDs include:

   i. poverty
   ii. crowded neighborhoods with high rates of drug use and infection
   iii. delays in seeking health care

G. Primary prevention strategies for STDs include:

   i. education about preventing spread of infection

H. Secondary prevention strategies include:

   i. early detection
   ii. effective treatment of early-stage STDs
   iii. effective case management

I. Tertiary prevention strategies include appropriate long-term treatment and management of chronic conditions for optimal outcomes. These are especially important for viral STDs.

2. Viral Sexually Transmitted Diseases. STDs in this category are caused by a viral infectious agent. There is no cure for viral sexually transmitted diseases, although in some cases the virus can be controlled.

   A. **Acquired Immunodeficiency Syndrome (AIDS)**

    i. AIDS is caused by infection with the **human immunodeficiency virus (HIV),** a retrovirus that attacks the body's infection-fighting cells. The infected person becomes vulnerable to a range of diseases. HIV/AIDS ultimately causes destruction of the immune system.

    ii. Vulnerable populations:

       a. anyone having unprotected sex or sharing needles with infected persons

       b. babies born to HIV-positive mothers

       c. people exposed to blood products or tissues of infected persons

    iii. Primary prevention of AIDS:

       a. avoid sexual intercourse or maintain mutually monogamous sexual relationship with uninfected person

       b. avoid sharing needles

    iv. Secondary prevention:

       a. low-cost testing, especially for pregnant women

       b. drug treatment facilities

       c. protecting health care workers from exposure

    v. Tertiary prevention:

       a. connecting clients with appropriate support agencies

       b. informing clients of new treatments that improve outcomes

    vi. Treatment of AIDS includes protease inhibitors and reverse transcriptase inhibitors, designed to keep the virus from reproducing and destroying disease-fighting cells.

B. **Human Papillomavirus.** The human papillomavirus (HPV) infects the anal and genital area, and is found in an increasing number of people in the United States.

    i. HPV is often asymptomatic.

    ii. Some people with HPV develop genital warts, which are highly contagious.

    iii. The most vulnerable population is young people; they are often infected but do not know it.

    iv. People who develop genital warts are at a higher risk of developing cancer of the cervix, anus, penis, and vulva.

    v. Treatment of HPV consists of removing warts through chemical applications, cryotherapy, laser, or electrosurgery to reduce the chance of transmission.

    vi. Removal of the warts, however, is not a cure: an outbreak can reoccur months or years later.

C. **Herpes Simplex Virus 2.** The herpes simplex virus 2 (HSV-2) is also known as genital herpes.

      i. HSV-2 is a contagious, chronic infection that causes sores in and around the vaginal area or anal area, on the penis, and on the buttocks or thighs.

     ii. Symptoms include:
        a. burning sensation in the genitals
        b. low back pain
        c. pain on urination
        d. flu-like symptoms may accompany the initial outbreak

    iii. The most vulnerable populations are sexually active people and newborns infected by contact with lesions during birth. Cesarean section delivery may be used to avoid exposing the newborn to genital lesions.

    iv. There is no known cure for HSV-2 infection. Antiviral medications can reduce duration and symptoms of an outbreak.

3. Bacterial Sexually Transmitted Diseases. STDs in this category are caused by a bacterial infectious agent. Many bacterial sexually transmitted diseases are treatable with antibiotics, although strains of drug-resistant bacterial STDs are becoming more common.

  A. **Chlamydia.** The most frequently reported STD in the United States. Its symptoms can include vaginal discharge, burning on urination, and pain during intercourse for women, and itching and burning around the penis for men.

      i. The most vulnerable populations are sexually active people. Chlamydia infection often has no symptoms, and those with the infection may pass it on to others without knowing it. Newborns may also be infected during delivery.

     ii. Treatment is a regimen of antibiotics. Treatment for gonorrhea is generally given at the same time, since infection with both diseases often occurs.

  B. **Syphilis.** This STD can lead to serious debilitating disease if left untreated.

      i. Syphilis has three stages:
        a. primary: characterized by a painless lesion at site of entry of bacterium
        b. secondary: characterized by infectious lesions and flu-like symptoms
        c. tertiary: If left untreated, syphilis progresses to the tertiary stage, which includes mental deterioration and other complications.

     ii. Vulnerable populations include sexually active persons, newborns infected during birth, and women (who may not have symptoms).

    iii. Syphilis is treated with penicillin.

C. **Gonorrhea.** This STD is a frequently occurring infection that affects over a million Americans each year. It often occurs in tandem with chlamydia.

    i. Symptoms include discharge and pain on urination for men. Many women do not have symptoms, or infection presents only as mild discomfort during urination.

    ii. Vulnerable populations include:

        a. sexually active people (gonorrhea can infect the genitals, throat, or anus)

        b. newborns during birth

        c. children who are sexually abused

        d. anyone who has sex with a **carrier,** a person who harbors the infectious agent without ever showing symptoms of the disease

    iii. Treatment is a course of antibiotics. Some gonorrhea strains have developed resistance to antibiotics.

D. **Trichomoniasis.** Commonly called "trich," this STD affects 2 to 3 million Americans each year. Symptoms in women generally include a greenish-yellow vaginal discharge with a foul odor, as well as burning and painful urination. Men may have mild irritation or tingling sensation in the penis.

    i. Vulnerable populations include all sexually active people, especially women. Trichomoniasis often occurs along with gonorrhea and may facilitate HIV infection.

    ii. Treatment is a dose of metronidazole. Screening and treatment for other STDs is recommended on finding trichomoniasis.

4. The role of the community health nurse in preventing sexually transmitted diseases

A. **Primary prevention** strategies:

    i. educating health care providers and the public about STDs, symptoms, treatments, and preventing transmission

    ii. educating people about risk factors and encouraging safer sex practices

B. **Secondary prevention** strategies:

    i. early detection and treatment of infection

    ii. partner notification to prevent further spread

    iii. screening pregnant women to prevent spread to fetus/newborn

C. **Tertiary prevention** strategies: minimizing and managing effects of chronic infections such as herpes, HIV, and untreated syphilis

5. The community health nurse needs to ensure that all educational materials and delivery of information should take into account the **cultural attitudes** surrounding sex and sexuality, making sure that materials and information are culturally appropriate.

REVIEW ACTIVITIES

Questions

1. Which of the following statements is true about sexually transmitted diseases (STDs) in the United States?

    a.   They seldom have any serious effects on health.

    b.   They make up half of the most frequently reported diseases.

    c.   Media messages have little impact on the prevention of STDs.

    d.   They can be cured with proper treatment.

2. Which of the following environmental factors contribute to the spread of STDs?

    a.   immunization

    b.   notification of sexual partners

    c.   education

    d.   poverty

3. Effective case management and treatment for STDs in the early stages are examples of:

    a.   environmental factors

    b.   primary prevention strategies

    c.   secondary prevention strategies

    d.   long-term strategies

4. STDs that have a viral infectious agent are:

    a.   AIDS, chlamydia, and gonorrhea

    b.   HPV, HSV-2, and HIV/AIDS

    c.   syphilis, gonorrhea, and herpes

    d.   none of the above

5. Which of the following statements about human papillomavirus (HPV) is true?

    a.   All people with HPV will develop genital warts.

    b.   Removing genital warts through cryotherapy or laser cures HPV infection.

    c.   People with genital warts from HPV are more likely to develop cancer of the cervix, anus, or penis.

    d.   The most vulnerable population is people over 50.

6. STDs that have a bacterial infectious agent are:

    a.   chlamydia, gonorrhea, and syphilis

    b.   gonorrhea, syphilis, and herpes

    c.   trichomoniasis and HIV

    d.   all of the above

7. A person diagnosed with chlamydia should also be screened for which disease that often occurs in tandem?

    a.   HIV

    b.   syphilis

    c.   gonorrhea

    d.   HPV

8. Symptoms of the tertiary stage of syphilis include:

    a.   mental deterioration

    b.   flu-like symptoms

    c.   painless lesion at the site of infection

    d.   painful urination

9. Populations vulnerable to gonorrhea include all of the following except:

    a.   sexually abused children

    b.   newborns

    c.   sexually active people

    d.   carriers

10. Which of the following STDs is thought to facilitate HIV infection?

    a.   gonorrhea

    b.   syphilis

    c.   trichomoniasis

    d.   chlamydia

Critical-Thinking Questions

1. A teenage couple that comes to your clinic believes that they can protect themselves against STDs by using oral or anal intercourse rather than penis/vagina intercourse. What are the primary, secondary, or tertiary prevention strategies that need to be implemented for these clients?

2. A male client complains of painful urination. He says "of course" when you ask if he is sexually active. What sexually transmitted diseases should he be screened for? What social or cultural factors may come into play with this client?

3. Name the most vulnerable populations for the following STDs:
   • AIDS
   • herpes simplex virus 2
   • chlamydia
   • syphilis
   • gonorrhea
Which vulnerable populations do they all have in common?

Discussion Questions

1. What STD education resources are available in your community? How do most people get information about the occurrence or prevention of STDs?

2. What is the most frequently occurring STD in your community? What population (age, ethnicity) has the highest rate of infection in your community?

3. For a population of your choice in your community, identify the primary, secondary, and tertiary prevention strategies in place for combating the spread of HIV/AIDS.

References

Allison, K. C. (1996). *American Medical Association complete guide to women's health.* New York: Random House.

Aral, S. O., et al. (1999). Sexual mixing patterns in the spread of gonococcal and chlamydial infections. *Am J Public Health, 89*(6), 825–833.

Brown, E. J., & Simpson, E. M. (2000). Comprehensive STD/HIV prevention education targeting US adolescents: Review of an ethical dilemma and proposed ethical framework. *Nurs Ethics, 7*(4), 339–349.

Coombes, R. (2000). Return of the dirty dozen: Sexually transmitted infections. *Nurs
Times, 96*(36), 12–13.

Hilton, B. A., Thompson, R., Moore-Dempsey, L., & Hutchinson, K. (2001). Urban
outpost nursing: The nature of the nurses' work in the AIDS Prevention Street
Nurse Program. *Public Health Nurs, 18*(4), 273–280.

Jones, K., & Roberts, A. (1999). Gonorrhea: The return. *Nurs Times, 95*(40), 54–55.

Logan, S. L., Freeman, E. M. (Eds.). (2000). *Healthcare in the black community: Empowerment, knowledge, skills, and collectivism.* New York: Haworth Press.

McDermott-Webster, M. (1999). Hospital extra: The HPV epidemic: Human papillomavirus infection. *Am J Nurs, 99*(3), 24L, 24N.

Rawlins, S. (2001). Nonviral sexually transmitted infections. *JOGNN, 30*(3), 324–331.

Ryan, C., & Futterman, D. (1998). *Lesbian and gay youth.* New York: Columbia University Press.

Schoeberlein, D. (2000). *EveryBody™: Preventing HIV and other sexually transmitted diseases among young teens.* Carbondale, CO: RAD Education Programs. http://
www.preventaids.net

Signorielli, N. (1993). *Mass media images and impact on health.* Westport, CT: Greenwood Press.

Thomas, D. J. (2001). Sexually transmitted viral infections: Epidemiology and treatment. *JOGNN, 30*(3), 22–23.

Zurlinden, J. (1999). Up close & clinical: Living with herpes. *Nurs Spectrum, 12*(18),
17.

Web Sites

Association of Nurses in AIDS Care (ANAC)
http://www.anacnet.org/

Journal of the American Sexually Transmitted Diseases Association
http://www.stdjournal.com

National Center for HIV, STD, and TB Prevention
http://www.cdc.gov/nchstp/dstd/dstdp.htm

NIAID Fact Sheet
http://www.niaid.nih.gov/factsheet/stdinfo.htm

Sexually Transmitted Diseases: Medline Plus Health Information
http://www.nlm.nih.gov/medlineplus/sexuallytransmitteddiseases.htm

World Health Organization: HIV/AIDS and Sexually Transmitted Infections
http://www/who.int/HIV_AIDS/

CHAPTER 12

CHRONIC ILLNESS

INTRODUCTION

A major population that community health nurses work with is composed of individuals living with a chronic illness or condition. This chapter examines the nurse's role in health promotion and disease prevention for those suffering from chronic illness.

KEY POINTS

1. **Chronic illness** is an altered health state that is not curable by simple medical procedures or by a short course of medical therapy.

    A. Chronic illness affects all age groups, not just the elderly.
    B. Chronic illness occurs across all racial and ethnic groups and all socioeconomic categories.
    C. Chronic illness affects family and community as well as the client.

2. According to the National Center for Health Statistics, chronic conditions with the highest prevalence rates in the United States are:

   A. orthopedic impairments
   B. chronic sinusitis
   C. arthritis
   D. high blood pressure
   E. hay fever/allergies
   F. hearing impairments
   G. heart disease
   H. chronic bronchitis
   I. asthma
   J. headache

3. The community health nurse's role in health promotion and disease prevention for chronic illness is essential. The nurse can help clients deal with the impacts of chronic disease, which include

   A. physical: such as altered health status, pain, disability
   B. psychological and spiritual: such as depression, isolation, loss of role in community, feeling of being punished or singled out
   C. economic: cost of care and supplies; loss of earning potential

4. The nurse's role focuses on different levels of prevention, with the most emphasis on preventing disease before it begins, rather than treating disease after it occurs.

5. **Primary prevention.** This first level of prevention seeks to alter risk factors before disease has begun. Primary prevention actions can include:

   A. modifying environmental or lifestyle **risk factors** (such as smoking, dietary fat, obesity)
   B. disease **prevention strategies** such as immunization
   C. **health education** such as teaching benefits of self-care (nutrition, exercise, adequate sleep, stress reduction)
   D. Principles of **empowerment** are essential to community health nursing.

      i. Empowerment assumes that people know themselves best.
      ii. As a result, they can effectively identify their own problems and the solutions to those problems more effectively than can an outside party.

6. **Secondary prevention.** The second level of prevention focuses on early disease detection and treatment. Secondary prevention strategies include:

A. screening for risk factors that can lead to chronic illness, such as cholesterol, blood pressure, and cancer screenings
B. detecting diseases with insidious onset
C. identifying populations at risk and using risk modification strategies

7. **Tertiary prevention.** The third level of prevention focuses on rehabilitation and restoration after illness has occurred. Tertiary prevention strategies include:

A. preventing complications associated with illnesses through regular examinations
B. addressing physical and psychosocial challenges associated with disease
C. helping people with chronic disease find appropriate support and resources in the community
D. providing assessment, planning, and interventions as part of a care team
E. being aware of cultural or ethnic perspectives about illness, healing modalities, and the like

8. **Healthy People 2010** is a survey by the U.S. Department of Health and Human Services used to measure the health of the U.S. population from 2000 to 2010. Goals include increasing the quality and years of healthy life and eliminating health disparities among different segments of the population.

9. The survey follows a variety of public health indicators and seeks information and understanding about the interplay of social and individual responsibility for health and the impact of these factors on public health.

10. Healthy People 2010 targets the following areas as ones that can affect chronic or long-term illness and disability:

A. lack of regular physical activity
B. overweight and obesity
C. tobacco use
D. substance abuse
E. irresponsible sexual behavior
F. mental illness
G. injury and violence
H. poor environmental quality
I. lack of immunizations

REVIEW ACTIVITIES

Questions

1. Which of the following statements about chronic illness is true?
   a. The community health nurse can do little to prevent chronic illness in a population.
   b. It is curable when the correct medical therapy is identified.
   c. Very few people in the United States are impacted by chronic illness.
   d. Nursing emphasis consists of preventing chronic illness before it occurs.

2. Primary prevention strategies for a chronic illness such as heart disease could include:
   a. modifying risk factors such as obesity or high-fat diet
   b. implementing disease prevention strategies such as regular aerobic exercise
   c. teaching people about healthy diet and exercise
   d. all of the above

3. The principle of empowerment can best be defined as:
   a. a way to place the responsibility for health care on clients
   b. recognizing that people can identify their own problems and solutions
   c. having clients choose between traditional and alternative health care
   d. making sure that the client is strengthened by the nurse's input

4. An example of a secondary prevention strategy for chronic illness would include which of the following?
   a. showing a client who has had a stroke how to walk with a cane
   b. conducting blood pressure screenings at the local mall
   c. helping people with diabetes find a support group and affordable monitoring supplies
   d. immunizing a client against influenza

5. An effective tertiary prevention strategy for a client with a significant hearing impairment would be:
   a. enrolling the client in a book group to avoid social isolation
   b. providing information on a company that makes lights that flash when the telephone rings
   c. insisting the client get hearing aids
   d. talking louder

6. According to the Healthy People 2010 survey, which of the following areas affect chronic illness?
   a. physical activity

b. use of tobacco and alcohol
c. the quality of a person's living environment
d. all of the above

Critical-Thinking Questions

1. For a client with insulin-dependent diabetes, identify the physical, psychological/spiritual, and economic impacts of the chronic illness on the client's life.

2. For the client in question 1, what are some of the prevention strategies available to assist this client in living with chronic illness?

3. How can the concept of empowerment be applied to a client with asthma?

Discussion Questions

1. In the client population you work with, or in your community, what are the most frequently occurring chronic illnesses?

2. In your community, how does a chronic illness such as high blood pressure affect
    • individuals
    • families
    • communities

3. In your community, which chronic diseases are most effectively addressed in the media? Do the media messages focus primarily on prevention? Detection? Support or services? Describe an example of an effective media campaign for a chronic illness in your community.

4. Identify some of the alternative, complementary, or culturally-based healing modalities practiced by populations in your community. Are these modalities generally accepted or rejected by the traditional health care community?

References

Bova, C. (2001). Adjustment to chronic illness among HIV-infected women. *J Nurs Sch, 33*(3), 217–223.

Braithwaite, R. L., Taylor, S. E., & Austin, J. N. (2000). *Building health coalitions in the black community*. Thousand Oaks, CA: Sage.

Brown, R. T. (1999). *Cognitive aspects of chronic illness in children*. New York: Guilford.

Champagne, D. (Ed.). (1999). *Contemporary Native American cultural issues*. Walnut Creek, CA: AltaMira Press.

Chesla, C. A., & Rungreangkulkij, S. (2001). Nursing research on family processes in chronic illness in ethnically diverse families: A decade review. *J Fam Nurs, 7*(3), 230–243.

Eliopoulous, C. (1997). *Gerontological nursing* (4th ed.). Philadelphia: Lippincott.

Henderson, A., & Champlin, S. (Eds.). (1998). *Promoting teen health: Linking schools, health organizations, and community*. Thousand Oaks, CA: Sage.

Hirschfelder, A. B. (1998). *The encyclopedia of smoking and tobacco*. Phoenix, AZ: Oryx Press.

Izenberg, N. (Ed.). (2000). *Human diseases and conditions*. New York: Charles Scribner's Sons.

Koch,T., & Kralik, D. (2001). Chronic illness: Reflections on a community-based action research programme. *J Adv Nurs, 36*(1), 23–31.

Miller, J. F. (2000). *Coping with chronic illness: Overcoming powerlessness*. Philadelphia: F. Davis.

Negidjon, B. M., & Sowers, K. W. (Eds.). (2000). *A nurse's guide to cancer care*. Philadelphia: Lippincott, Williams & Wilkins.

Nicassio, P. M., & Smith, T. W. (Eds.). (1998). *Managing chronic illness: A biopsychosocial perspective*. Washington, DC: American Psychological Association.

Paterson, B. (2001). Myth of empowerment in chronic illness. *J Adv Nurs, 34*(5), 574–581.

Wallace, H. M. (Ed.). (1997). *Mosby's guide to children with disabilities and chronic illness*. St. Louis, MO: Mosby.

Web Sites

American Cancer Society
http://www.cancer.org/

American Diabetes Association
http://www.diabetes.org/

American Heart Association
http://www.americanheart.org/

American Lung Association: Quitting Smoking Index
http://www.lungusa.org/tobacco/

Center for Research on Chronic Illness (CRCI), funded by the National Institute of Nursing Research
http://www.unc.edu/depts/crci

Chronic Illness: Nursing References (links to National Library of Medicine, Martindale's Virtual Nursing Guide, U.S. Department of Health and Human Services, National Institute of Nursing Research, etc.)
http://www.nursingnet.org/nr.htm

Hypertension Network (consumer information)
http://www.bloodpressure.com

National Cancer Institute
http://www.nci.nih.gov/

Tobacco Cessation Guidelines
http://www.surgeongeneral.gov/tobacco

Women and Heart Disease
http://www.cdc.gov/nccdphp/cvd/womensatlas/

Yale School of Nursing: Center for Excellence in Chronic Illness Care
http://www.info.med.yale.edu/nursing/centers/centers_chronic.html

13

MENTAL ILLNESS

KEY TERMS

community-based care	rapport
deinstitutionalization	respect
disaster	secondary prevention
disaster response	suicide
empathy	tertiary prevention
mental disorder	trust
primary prevention	

INTRODUCTION

There are many settings in which community health nurses provide services to people with mental illness. This chapter explores the common conditions a nurse might encounter working in a community practice, and the nurse's role in prevention and health maintenance.

KEY POINTS

1. The American Psychiatric Association (1994) defines **mental disorder** as "clinically significant behavior or psychological syndrome or pattern that occurs in an individual and is associated with present distress . . . or dis-

ability . . . with a significantly increased risk of suffering, death, pain, disability, or an important loss of freedom."

2. The way society deals with people with mental disorders or **mental illness** is a complex combination of political, economic, and cultural influences. The key current factors are:

    A.   mental health reform, with emphasis on:

        i.   **community-based care** such as day and evening programs
       ii.   halfway houses to transition between inpatient and outpatient care
      iii.   partial hospitalization programs
      iv.   emergency services

    B.   **deinstitutionalization**

        i.   began in the 1970s
       ii.   significant numbers of people from public mental hospitals are discharged to the community
      iii.   process assumes that support services for mentally ill people will be available so that they can function outside the institutional setting
      iv.   results have been mixed, especially given lack of appropriate community-based services in many areas

    C.   less coverage by private insurers for mental illness and substance abuse, compared with coverage provided for physical illness
    D.   consumer activism and involvement in advocating for effective services for people with mental illness

3. Key components of the community health nurse's relationship with people with mental disorders are:

    A.   **trust:** being consistent, respectful, and honest with the person with mental illness
    B.   building **rapport:** showing the person with mental illness that she or he is important and valuable
    C.   **respect:** accepting the person with mental illness nonjudgmentally
    D.   **empathy:** ability to understand that clients' perceptions are real to them, thus validating their experiences

4. The main categories of mental disorders or conditions that a community health nurse will encounter are:

    A.   anxiety
    B.   depression (including those who are suicidal)

C. schizophrenia
D. bipolar disorder
E. clients who have experienced violence or abuse

5. There are many settings in which community health nurses provide services to people with mental illness, including:

A. as part of multidisciplinary team or care providers, in a number of locations:

    i. shelters
    ii. food programs
    iii. senior centers
    iv. prisons
    v. primary care clinics
    vi. workplace employee assistance programs
    vii. cultural and neighborhood centers
    viii. private homes

B. as part of a network of supervised living settings that allows transition from institutional living to independent living such as

    i. halfway houses
    ii. group homes

C. providing ongoing health promotion and illness prevention for persons with mental illness

6. The goals of prevention in working with people with mental illness are to decrease onset, duration, and disability associated with mental illness.

A. **Primary prevention** strategies include:

    i. preventing onset of mental health disorders through education, especially targeting at-risk groups
    ii. educating—for example, teaching parenting skills, effects of alcohol and drugs
    iii. developing support systems
    iv. offering crisis intervention after stressful events.

B. **Secondary prevention** strategies include:

    i. early identification and treatment of illness or disorder to reduce cases in the at-risk population and shorten length of illness or episode
    ii. ongoing assessment of high-risk infants and children
    iii. provision of access to counseling, medication administration, suicide prevention, and case management

C. **Tertiary prevention** strategies include:

    i. reducing the effects caused by severe mental illness by addressing the social, medical, and psychiatric needs of ill persons
    ii. teaching daily living skills and case management

7. Suicidal clients

A. The symptoms of **suicide** may mimic physical illness.
B. At-risk populations are white, African American, Latino, and Native American males.
C. Other at-risk groups include:

    i. gay and lesbian youth
    ii. runaways
    iii. cult and gang members
    iv. people with a history of family violence
    v. people diagnosed with severe or terminal disease

8. Community **disaster response.** A **disaster** is a severe disruption that exceeds the coping skills and abilities of the affected community.

A. Anything that has a serious impact on the community is considered a disaster.
B. Some disasters are massive in scale (war, hurricanes, terrorist attack, and so on).
C. Some disasters are on a smaller scale (violence involving members of the community, the death of a person central to the community).
D. Community health nurses can be key in community planning efforts to prepare for disaster response
E. Disaster response for any community should include:

    i. preparing for people's emotional responses to disaster
    ii. ensuring that vital services for vulnerable people and caregivers are maintained

9. Legal aspects of nursing care for clients with mental disorders. The community health nurse should be aware that people with mental disorders have a legal right to the following:

A. right to treatment: including examination, treatment plan, and review
B. confidentiality: information cannot be revealed without the client's consent
C. consent: the person with mental illness has to agree to treatment (unless certified as incompetent to do so)
D. right to refuse treatment: the person with mental illness can refuse treatments such as medications (unless certified as incompetent to do so)

E.   right to hearing: the person with a mental disorder has the right to a hearing to determine competence; used in cases of involuntary commitment for clients considered dangerous to themselves or others

REVIEW ACTIVITIES

Questions

1. Which of the following would be considered community-based care for a person with a mental disorder?
    a.   residential program at a private treatment center
    b.   group therapy program each evening from 7 to 9 at the local mental health center
    c.   psychiatric inpatient wing of the local hospital
    d.   none of the above

2. Which of the following is true about deinstitutionalization?
    a.   It seldom happens in U.S. mental health care.
    b.   It is used only for a small segment of the people formerly living in public mental health hospitals.
    c.   It assumes that community-based services are readily available to people who have mental illness.
    d.   It coincides with increased coverage by insurance companies.

3. A community health nurse would be likely to work with people with mental disorders in which of the following settings?
    a.   shelters and food programs
    b.   neighborhood centers and clinics
    c.   prisons
    d.   all of the above

4. Building rapport with a client with a mental disorder is best defined as:
    a.   being consistent and honest
    b.   accepting the person and avoiding judgment
    c.   showing that the person is valued
    d.   none of the above

5. An example of a primary prevention strategy for working with a person with a mental disorder would be:
    a.   quickly identifying a person who is schizophrenic
    b.   providing education on drug and alcohol abuse to a teenager whose family has a history of alcoholism and depression

   c.   teaching daily living skills to a person who is suicidal

   d.   monitoring medication prescribed to alleviate severe anxiety

6. Which of the following would be considered at risk for suicide?

   a.   African American women

   b.   runaway teens

   c.   Asian males

   d.   children in an inner-city reading program

7. Which of the following best defines disaster?

   a.   an event that causes minimal disruption to everyday life

   b.   an event that exceeds the coping skills of the community it affects

   c.   an event that is always large in scale

   d.   an event that always involves natural occurrences such floods or hurricanes

8. The concept of consent for a person with a mental disorder means:

   a.   the nurse must agree to treat the client

   b.   people with mental disorders are not required to consent to treatment

   c.   the people providing care must ensure that the client agrees to receive the care

   d.   the nurse must agree not to reveal information about the client

Critical-Thinking Questions

1. Describe secondary prevention strategies that would be appropriate for the client of a food bank who will accept only canned vegetables because all other foods, according to him, "have been poisoned."

2. Describe the primary prevention strategies that a community health nurse could provide for occupants of a city jail. What mental disorders might the nurse be likely to encounter?

3. You are evaluating a Latino male who has just left a seven-year relationship with his girlfriend. He says that the relationship was sometimes "wild" and that they fought verbally and physically. Should he be considered at-risk for suicide? Why or why not? What other mental disorders or distress might he be at risk for?

Discussion Questions

1. What community-based mental health resources are available in your community? How do people learn about them? Do you think that your community's resources are adequate or inadequate? Why or why not?

2. Identify a population in your community that is at risk for suicide.

3. In the past three years, has your community experienced a disaster that disrupted its coping skills? Describe the type of disaster it was (large or smaller scale, act of nature, tragedy involving a member of the community) and how it impacted your community.

4. What resources are available in your community to help people cope with disasters? How do you access these resources?

References

Ahern, L., & Fisher, D. (2001). Recovery at your own PACE (personal assistance in community existence). *J Psychosoc Nurs Ment Health Serv, 39*(4), 22–32.

Barr, W., Cotterill, L., & Hoskins, A. (2001). Improving community mental health nurse targeting of people with severe and enduring mental illness: Experiences from one English health district. *J Adv Nurs, 34*(1), 117–127.

Barry, P. (2001). *Mental health & mental illness* (7th ed.). Philadelphia: Lippincott.

Chien, W., Kam, C., & Lee, I. F. (2001). An assessment of the patients' needs in mental health education. *J Adv Nurs, 34*(3), 304–311.

Corbett, R. W., & Mashburn, D. (2000). Nurses in disaster. *Excellence Clin Pract, 1*(3), 1, 3.

Coyle, B. (2001). Suicide and the young. *Community Pract, 74*(1), 8–9.

Diagnostic and statistical manual of mental disorders. DSM-IV-TR (4th ed.). Washington, DC: American Psychiatric Association.

Forrester, M. (2001). Managing depression in the community. *Ment Health Nurs, 21*(5), 23–25.

Gorlin, R. A. (Ed.). (1999). *Codes of professional responsibility*. Washington, DC: Bureau of Professional Affairs.

Hanlon, J. (2001). Time for a change: The practice nurse and preventing mental illness. *Pract Nurse, 21*(5), 20, 22, 25.

Horsfall, J. (2001). *Interpersonal nursing for mental health*. New York: Springer.

Kadum, D. (2000). NT practice solutions: How to protect patients who are at risk of self-harm or suicide. *Nurs Times, 97*(30), 44.

Kupers, T. A. (1999). *Prison madness: The mental health crisis behind bars and what we must do about it*. San Francisco: Jossey-Bass.

Moore, A. (2001). Chaos theory: Disaster relief nursing. *Nurs Stand, 15*(31), 14–16.

Schneidman, E. S. (2001). *Comprehending suicide: Landmarks in 20th century suicidology*. Washington, DC: American Psychological Association.

White, L. (2001). *Foundations of nursing: Caring for the whole person*. Clifton Park, NY: Delmar Learning.

Web Sites

Anxiety Disorders Association of America
http://www.adaa.org/

Anxiety Disorders Education Program
http://www.nimh.nih.gov/anxiety/

Association for Death Education and Counseling
http://www.adec.org

Depression: National Institute of Mental Health
http://www.nimh.nih.gov/publicat/depressionmenu.cfm

International Society for Mental Health Online
http://www.ismho.org/

Issues in Mental Health Nursing
http://www.tandf.co.uk/journals/tf/01612840.html

Journal of Psychiatric and Mental Health Nursing
http://www.blackwell-science.com/products/journals/jpmhn.htm

Journal of Psychosocial Nursing
http://www.slackinc.com/allied/jpn/jpnhome.htm

National Institute of Mental Health
http://www.nimh.gov/

National Mental Health Association
http://www.nmha.org/

Online Dictionary of Mental Health
http://www.shef.ac.uk/~psych/psychotherapy/

Substance Abuse and Mental Health Services Administration (SAMHSA)
http://www.samhsa.org/

CHAPTER 14

HOMELESSNESS

homelessness
peripheral vascular disease
primary prevention

secondary prevention
tertiary prevention
thermatoregulatory disorders

INTRODUCTION

Homelessness is a growing problem that has a profound impact on the individuals, families, and communities it touches. Community health nurses need to be aware of the constellation of factors that surround homelessness in order to effectively combat the problem. This chapter looks at the changing face of homelessness, the causes, and several prevention strategies.

KEY POINTS

1. According to the Stewart B. McKinney Act (1994), a person is considered homeless if he or she

   A. lacks a fixed, regular, and adequate nighttime residence
   B. has a primary nighttime residence that is

      i. a supervised shelter designed to provide temporary living accommodations
      ii. an institution that provides temporary residence

      iii. public or private place not designed to be used as a regular sleeping place for humans

2. The demographics of the homeless population are as follows:

  A. age: 51 percent are between ages 31 and 50; children under 18 comprise 25 percent of urban homeless
  B. gender: more males than females
  C. families with children: the fastest-growing segment of the homeless population in the past 10 years; estimated at 38 percent of urban homeless
  D. location: Homeless people are found in both urban and rural settings.
  E. ethnicity: U.S. Conference of Mayors (1998) found that 49 percent of homeless populations were African American, 32 percent Caucasian, 12 percent Hispanic, 4 percent Native American, and 3 percent Asian.
  F. Ethnic makeup of a homeless population likely varies according to geographic region.

3. The causes of homelessness are a complex combination of a variety of factors, including:

  A. economic
  B. social
  C. personal
  D. political

4. Community health nurses need to be aware of the constellation of factors that surround homelessness, including:

  A. cultural and religious factors:

     i. family structures
    ii. attitudes regarding sex and marriage
   iii. domestic violence
   iv. shift from rural to urban living

  B. social and economic factors:

     i. lack of affordable housing
    ii. minimum-wage service sector
   iii. female-headed households
   iv. loss of government benefits
    v. high unemployment

  C. sexual orientation

D. legal status:

    i. immigration status
    ii. marital status
    iii. mental status
    iv. veterans

E. criminal record
F. language barriers
G. poor literacy skills
H. deinstitutionalization

5. Homelessness has a profound effect on individuals, families, and the community. The community health nurse's knowledge of all these aspects is crucial for effective interventions.

6. Even though homelessness is a community problem, many communities do not want to deal with it.

7. Private and public programs are available to assist homeless populations. Community health nurses need to know resources in both areas.

8. Private-sector responses include shelters, soup kitchens and outreach vans, and day programs.

9. Daily contact between homeless people and community health nurses can build trust, which allows nurses to practice primary prevention and intervention before health crises develop.

A. Increasingly, programs are able to focus on primary and secondary prevention rather than just tertiary prevention.
B. **Primary prevention:** preventing people from becoming homeless and preventing illness in those who are. This can include:

    i. for people at risk of homelessness: assessment of risks, bolstering support systems, and impacting political processes and decisions that might put marginal populations at risk
    ii. for people who are homeless: helping ensure safe living arrangements, sanitary and nutritious food, immunizations, and education programs regarding specific health threats such as TB and HIV

C. **Secondary prevention:** early detection and prevention of disability. Secondary prevention strategies can include:

    i. screening for TB and administering prophylactic medications
    ii. screening for other conditions such as high blood pressure, cancer, diabetes

    iii.   monitoring and treatment of wounds, to prevent infection
    iv.   monitoring prescribed medications

D. **Tertiary prevention:** treatment to minimize disability once illness has
    occurred. Tertiary prevention strategies can include:

    i.   providing discharge planning that recognizes limited resources
    ii. helping clients negotiate support agencies and treatment plans
    iii. educating other health care providers about the particular chal-
         lenges that homeless people face

10. Health problems common in homeless populations:

A. Alcoholism or substance abuse
B. Mental illness
C. Trauma from battery or assault

    i.   can occur in shelters, on the street, or in accidents
    ii. homeless people are often reluctant to report these incidents or to
         seek treatment
    iii. sexual assault and battery is a major risk for homeless persons

D. Nutritional deficiencies

    i.   caused by the lack of a balanced diet, alcoholism or drug use, and
         prescription drug use
    ii. homeless people needing special diets for conditions such as dia-
         betes may find it extremely difficult to regulate their diet

E. **Peripheral vascular disease** caused by

    i.   no place to sit or elevate feet
    ii. exposure to dampness and temperature extremes
    iii. socks and shoes that do not fit
    iv. poor nutrition and other underlying health conditions may make
         peripheral vascular disease worse

F. **Thermatoregulatory disorders:** hypothermia or hyperthermia, due to

    i.   exposure
    ii. lack of proper clothing
    iii. alcohol and drug use
    iv. burns from fires used for warmth and structure fires

G. HIV/AIDS, due to

    i.   needle sharing
    ii. unprotected sex
    iii. sexual abuse
    iv. teens and women are populations at very high risk.

H. Infectious diseases

    i. Infections are easily spread in shelters and other congregate living facilities.

    ii. Homeless are more vulnerable due to poor nutrition, substance abuse, stress, chronic medical conditions, and increase in drug-resistant disease strains.

I. Infestations, such as lice or scabies, due to

    i. crowded living conditions

    ii. poor sanitation

    iii. reluctance to seek treatment or inability to maintain treatment

J. Childhood illnesses, due to

    i. lack of immunizations

    ii. environmental factors such as lead exposure

    iii. delay in receiving treatment

K. Chronic conditions, made worse by lack of supplies, lack of access to care, and lifestyle

REVIEW ACTIVITIES

Questions

1. Which of the following statements about homeless populations is true?
    a. There are more homeless women than men.
    b. Virtually no homelessness occurs in rural areas.
    c. More families with children are becoming homeless.
    d. The majority of homeless people in the United States are Hispanic.

2. A possible economic factor for people becoming homeless would be:
    a. getting divorced
    b. having a minimum-wage job
    c. being removed from public assistance
    d. all of the above

3. A single mother with three children has just lost her job. Her rent is past due and she is in danger of being evicted. An example of a primary prevention strategy that a community health nurse could provide would be:
    a. putting her in touch with the community resources such as subsidized housing

b. taking her to the local shelter before it fills up

c. making sure her children are screened for TB and pediculosis

d. giving her brochures on HIV infection and foot care

4. Which of the following is an example of a secondary prevention strategy for men living in an urban homeless shelter?

a. monitoring medicine prescribed for diabetes

b. checking their feet for blisters and infection

c. checking their blood pressure

d. all of the above

5. A new volunteer physician in the shelter in which you work as a community health nurse says, "Mr. Jones will never properly control his diabetes if he doesn't take his medicine and watch his diet." An appropriate response would be to

a. tell the physician you agree with her assessment

b. educate the physician that, for homeless people like Mr. Jones, controlling diet is extremely difficult

c. insist that the physician talk to Mr. Jones about his eating habits

d. do nothing

6. Homeless people often have which of these health problems?

a. trauma or injury

b. nutritional deficits

c. infectious diseases

d. all of the above

7. Homeless persons can develop peripheral vascular disease due to:

a. the fact that they do not walk around much

b. their feet get cold and damp in winter and hot in summer

c. they can sit down and put their feet up during the day since they do not work

d. poor personal hygiene

8. A homeless person who had been drinking wine and walking all day in a cold rain without a jacket would be at risk for:

a. catching a cold

b. thermatoregulatory disorder

c. HIV infection

d. mental illness

9. Which of the following is true about assault and homeless people?

a. Homeless people are at low risk for assault in shelters.

b. Homeless people will readily report an assault to the police.

c. Homeless people are at significant risk for sexual assault.

d. None of the above.

10. Which of these factors put a homeless person at increased risk for infectious diseases?

    a.   living in a shelter
    b.   presence of drug-resistant diseases such as TB
    c.   poor nutrition
    d.   all of the above

Critical-Thinking Questions

1. Discuss how low literacy and inability to speak English fluently could put an immigrant at risk for homelessness.

2. Name two economic and two social factors that would put a rural family at risk for homelessness. What cultural factors could lower this risk?

3. Discuss how mental illness and deinstitutionalization can contribute to homelessness.

4. Name three primary prevention strategies for people at risk for becoming homeless, and three strategies for people who have just become homeless.

Discussion Questions

1. What facilities are available for the homeless in your community? How do people access these resources?

2. What is the demographic makeup of the homeless population in your community? Primarily male? Family? Ethnic group?

3. What is your risk of becoming homeless? What resources would you draw on if tomorrow you woke up with no job and no housing?

4. What physical illnesses or disorders are specific to homeless people in your area? What are the greatest risks?

REFERENCES

Baumohj, J. B. (Ed.). (1996). *Homeless in America*. Phoenix: Oryx Press.

Bruya, M. A., Thiele, J. E., & Synoground, G. (2001). Use of a search model to enhance patient education in a clinical setting. *J Contin Educ Nurs, 32*(4), 165–170.

Carter, J. H., Cuvar, K., McSweeney, M., Storey, P. J., & Stockman, C. (2001) Health seeking behavior as an outcome of a homeless population. *Outcomes Manage Nurs Pract, 5*(3), 140–144.

Hatton, D. C., Kleffel, D., Bennett, S., & Gaffrey, J. (2001). Homeless women and children's access to health care: A paradox. *J Community Health Nurs, 18*(1), 25–34.

Hitchcock, J., Schubert, P., & Thomas, S. (1999). *Community health nursing: Caring in action*. Clifton Park, NY: Delmar Learning.

Kelly, E. (2001). Assessment of dietary intake of preschool children living in a homeless shelter. *Appl Nurs Res, 14*(3), 146–154.

Killon, C. M. (2000). Extending the extended family for homeless and marginally housed African American women. *Public Health Nurs, 17*(5), 346–354.

Kozol, J. (1988). *Rachel and her children: Homeless families in America*. New York: Crown Publishers.

Majka, G. (2001). A case management, education, and prevention program at a small emergency shelter for homeless men: One nurse's experience. *J Emerg Nurs, 27*(3), 255–259.

National Coalition for the Homeless. (1997). *Fact sheet #8: Health care and homelessness*. Washington, DC: National Coalition for the Homeless.

National Coalition for the Homeless. (1998). *Fact Sheet #3: Who is homeless?* Washington, DC: National Coalition for the Homeless.

Swanson, J. M., & Nies, M. A. (Eds.). (1997). *Community health nursing: Promoting the health of aggregates* (2nd ed.). Philadelphia: Saunders.

Wilk, J. (1999). Health care for the homeless: A model for nursing education. *Int Nurs Rev, 46*(6), 171.

Web Sites

Division of Tuberculosis Elimination: Management of Homeless TB Patients
http://www.cdc.gov/mchstp/tb/notes/TB_2_00/reb.htm

Healthcare for the Homeless Information Resource Center
www.hchirc.com

HIV and Homeless Shelters: Policy and Practice available at
http://www.aclu.org/issues/gay/hiv_homeless.html

Institute for Children and Poverty
http://www.homesforthehomeless.com/abouthfh.html

National Coalition for the Homeless
http://www.nationalhomeless.org/who.html

National Coalition for Homeless Veterans
http://www.nchv.org/

National Healthcare for the Homeless Council
http://www.nhchc.org/

Urban Institute
http://www.urban.org

CHAPTER
15

ADDICTION

at-risk populations
dual diagnoses
primary prevention
risk factors
secondary prevention

situational stressors
substance abuse
substance dependence
tertiary prevention

INTRODUCTION

Community health nurses are often the first to recognize that a substance dependence or abuse problem exists and are therefore on the front lines of preventing and treating substance abuse. This chapter discusses the definitions of substance abuse and dependence, the common risk factors for substance abuse, and the nurse's role in prevention and health maintenance.

KEY POINTS

1. **Substance dependence** and **substance abuse** are maladaptive patterns of using substances characterized by:

   A. increasing tolerance
   B. withdrawal symptoms if the substance is stopped

C. significant distress or impairment of life functions due to the substance use

2. Substances that can be abused include

A. alcohol
B. amphetamines
C. caffeine
D. cannabis
E. cocaine
F. hallucinogens
G. inhalants
H. nicotine
I. opioids
J. PCP or similar drug
K. sedatives or hypnotics
L. combinations of these substances

3. Community health nurses need to be familiar with populations at risk for substance abuse.

4. The most pervasive risk factor for substance abuse is poverty. Other **risk factors** include:

A. learned coping or adaptive behaviors that include substance use
B. social roles
C. genetic factors
D. age
E. race
F. socioeconomic class
G. occupation

4. The following are considered **at-risk populations:**

A. Women

  i. Women have different risk factors, addiction patterns, and treatment needs, and often have additional barriers to treatment, such as financial and logistical constraints.
  ii. Primary risk factors for women include:
    a. childhood physical and sexual abuse
    b. domestic violence
    c. a partner or spouse who is a substance abuser
  iii. It is estimated that at least 80 percent of women incarcerated for drug charges use substances to alleviate the effects of previous physical or sexual abuse.

iv. The community health nurse must establish an environment of safety in which women can seek treatment, especially women in abusive relationships.

v. Alcohol affects women differently than it does men.

vi. There is an increased risk to women's reproductive health due to substance abuse, especially heavy drinking.

vii. More of a stigma seems to exist for women substance abusers; they may be more harshly treated by the system. As a result they are often slower to seek treatment.

B. Elders

i. Alcohol and substance abuse in older populations often is not correctly diagnosed; other conditions may disguise substance abuse.

ii. Elders often begin abusing substances, especially alcohol, as a response to **situational stressors** such as retirement, loss of spouse, loss of independence, and the like.

iii. Aging changes the way the body metabolizes alcohol and other drugs; alcohol intake may also interact or interfere with prescription medicines.

iv. Chronic drinking by elderly persons can have serious health impacts and also increases risk for falls and fractures.

C. People with Mental Illness; Homeless People

i. Many people have **dual diagnoses** of mental illness and addiction.

ii. Mentally ill people may use alcohol or other substances to lessen the symptoms of their illness or to offset side effects of medications.

iii. Often facilities treat the identified mental illness but not the substance abuse, or vice versa.

iv. Homeless men and women who have substance abuse problems and mental illness are at highest risk for trauma, physical illness, and legal problems.

D. Gays and Lesbians

i. There is a high prevalence of alcoholism in the gay and lesbian community.

ii. Possible causes include stress related to homophobia, and alcohol-based social settings such as bars. No definitive studies have been done.

E. Health Professionals

i. Alcohol and drug abuse cases account for two-thirds of complaints brought to state nursing boards.

    ii. Possible reasons for high rates of substance abuse include:
      a. genetic factors
      b. high stress levels
      c. easy access to drugs
      d. belief that knowledge of substances will protect the user from addiction.

5. Primary prevention strategies include health promotion and disease prevention:

    A. recognizing the social and behavioral etiologies of addiction
    B. educating people about society's deeply rooted norms about smoking, alcohol consumption, and the like
    C. assessing the community's understanding or perception of the problem
    D. determining the highest-risk groups in a particular population

6. Education about substances and substance use and abuse needs to be culturally sensitive and appropriate. Education can take place in a variety of settings:

    A. school
    B. work
    C. clinics
    D. shelters
    E. private homes
    F. church
    G. through the neighborhood/on the streets

7. Secondary prevention strategies consist of early intervention:

    A. assessment of client situation (which requires forming alliance and trust)
    B. looking at all areas of clients' lives:

      i. environmental (neighborhood, family, support systems)
      ii. behavioral (coping mechanisms)
      iii. physical (health status, use of medications)
      iv. emotional (stress, mental illness, resilience)

    C. recognition that people with substance abuse, especially IV drug users, are at high risk for HIV infection as well as other needle-transmitted diseases such as hepatitis
    D. screening and prenatal care for pregnant women to prevent transmission or diseases to the child, or to prevent babies from being born addicted or with fetal alcohol syndrome

8. Tertiary prevention strategies include treating the illness to minimize its effects.

    A.   Interventions at this level may not be enough to meet the complex care needs of persons with illnesses resulting from substance or alcohol abuse such as cirrhosis, HIV/AIDS, emphysema, and cancer.

    B.   Treatment also needs to address the systemic effects due to long-term or chronic alcohol or substance abuse.

REVIEW ACTIVITIES

Questions

1. A sign of substance dependence or abuse would be:
  a. withdrawal symptoms if the substance is reduced or stopped
  b. decreased tolerance to the substance
  c. little impairment of life or function due to substance abuse
  d. presence of adaptive coping strategies

2. Which of the following is true about risk factors for substance abuse?
  a. Poverty has little bearing on whether people choose to use substances.
  b. Genetic factors play a role in substance abuse.
  c. Substance abuse is not affected by age, gender, or occupation.
  d. None of the above.

3. Which of the following statements about women and alcohol is true?
  a. It is generally easy for women to access treatment for alcohol or substance abuse.
  b. Alcohol has the same impact on men and women.
  c. A woman whose significant other is a substance abuser is at higher risk for substance abuse.
  d. There is no known link between women, substance abuse, and physical abuse.

4. Which of the following statements about elders and alcohol/substance abuse is most accurate?
  a. It is readily apparent if an elder person has been abusing substances or alcohol.
  b. Elders who abuse substances or alcohol often do so to alleviate stresses such as grief or isolation.
  c. Alcohol consumption has little or no impact on prescription medications that an elder person may take.
  d. Alcohol or substance use does not increase the risk of falling or accidents.

5. In addition to elders and women, which of the following populations are at significant risk for substance or alcohol abuse?
   a. people with mental disorders
   b. gays and lesbians
   c. health professionals
   d. all of the above

6. Which of the following statements about alcohol and substance use in the gay community is most accurate?
   a. Alcohol abuse is not related to homophobia or other social stresses experienced by gays and lesbians.
   b. There is an extremely low rate of alcoholism in the gay and lesbian community.
   c. Of all at-risk populations, gays and lesbians are at greatest risk for legal problems because of substance use.
   d. Alcohol-based social settings such as bars may impact the level of alcohol use, but no clear data are available.

7. Of the following, what is a possible reason for substance abuse among health professionals?
   a. It is more difficult for health professionals to get access to drugs.
   b. Health professionals think that because they know about substances they will not become addicted.
   c. Nursing and other ethics boards tend to act as if the problem does not exist.
   d. Most health professionals have dual diagnoses of mental illness and addiction.

8. Teaching elementary school children and their parents how media ads (such as Joe Camel) target young people and try to make smoking look "cool" is an example of a:
   a. tertiary prevention strategy
   b. secondary prevention strategy
   c. primary prevention strategy
   d. none of the above

9. Which of the following is an example of a secondary prevention strategy?
   a. educating young women about the consequences of alcohol abuse while pregnant
   b. treating a homeless man's kidney failure brought on by long-term alcohol abuse
   c. identifying young males living in poverty as at higher risk for substance use or abuse
   d. providing assessment for a woman in an abusive relationship, examining her living arrangement, how she copes with stress, and her physical status

Critical-Thinking Questions

1. You are performing an assessment on Mr. Quinn, a 75-year-old man, who lives alone. His wife of 44 years died two months ago. Mr. Quinn's son is concerned because his father has fallen twice in the past month and seems to be "getting kind of spacey." When you ask if Mr. Quinn uses alcohol, his son says, "Oh, he was a social drinker, when he and my mom went out. But he probably doesn't drink anymore." What is your assessment of Mr. Quinn's risk for alcohol abuse? Why?

2. You are beginning intervention with a 45-year-old homeless man with a history of mental illness. The shelter where he has been staying reports that he smells of alcohol when he returns to the shelter in the evening and has been acting increasingly erratic. What do you need to know about each of the following areas in the man's life to begin an effective intervention and secondary prevention?
   - environmental
   - behavioral
   - physical
   - emotional

3. Your patient is a 24-year-woman who has just been incarcerated. The charge was selling cocaine and amphetamines, which she says belonged to her boyfriend. As a community health nurse, you know the risk factors and treatment challenges that exist for women. Identify one possible:
   - primary prevention strategy
   - secondary prevention strategy
   - tertiary prevention strategy

4. What are your attitudes about people who abuse substances or alcohol? Does someone in your family abuse substances or alcohol? Could these factors impact how you work with this population? Why or why not?

5. In your opinion, should all health care workers undergo drug screening as a condition or employment? Why or why not? What are the advantages and disadvantages of drug screening of health professionals?

Discussion Questions

1. What groups in your community are at the highest risk for alcohol or substance abuse?

2. What resources are available to these populations? How do people find out about available resources?

3. Are any of the resources in your community targeted specifically to certain populations? Homeless, mentally ill, women, gay/lesbian?

4. How does the media in your community participate in educating people about substance or alcohol use or abuse? How effective are these strategies?

5. Describe an educational strategy that you have seen or heard for teaching children about:
- alcohol
- cocaine
- nicotine
- inhalants

Was the strategy effective or ineffective? Why or why not?

References

American Nurses Association. (1989). *Standards of addiction nursing practice with selected diagnoses and criteria*. Washington, DC: American Nurses Association.
Barry, P. (2001). *Mental health & mental illness* (7th ed.). Philadelphia: Lippincott.
Boys, A., Marsden, J., & Strang, J. (2001). Understanding reasons for drug use amongst young people: A functional perspective. *Health Educ Res, 16*(4), 457–469.

Brown, S. (1995). *Treating alcoholism*. San Francisco: Jossey-Bass.

Carson-Dewitt, R. (Ed.). (2001). *Encyclopedia of drugs, alcohol, and addictive behavior*. New York: Macmillan Reference.

Cooper, D. B., & Cooper, P. D. (2001). Helping people with alcohol problems. *Prof Nurs, 16*(8), 1276–1280.

Craft-Rosenberg, M., & Denehy, J. (Eds.). (2001). *Nursing interventions for infants, children and families*. Thousand Oaks, CA: Sage.

Daley, D., Moss, H., & Campbell, F. (1993). *Dual disorders*. Center City, MN: Hazelden Foundation.

Diagnostic and statistical manual of mental disorders. DSM-IV-TR (4th ed.). Washington, DC: American Psychiatric Association.

Henderson-Martin, B. (2001). No more surprises: Screening patients for alcohol abuse. *Am J Nurs, 100*(9), 26–33.

Jackson-Koku, G. (2001). Mental health, mental illness and substance misuse: A nursing challenge. *Br J Nurs, 10*(4), 242–246.

Kelly, P. J., Blacksin, B., & Mason, E. (2001). Factors affecting substance abuse treatment completion for women. *Issues Ment Health Nurs, 22*(3), 287–304.

Lindenberg, C. S., Solorzano, R. M., Vilaro, F. M., & Westbrook, R. O. (2001). Challenges and strategies for conducting intervention research with culturally diverse populations. *J Transcult Nurs, 12*(2), 132–139.

Meyers, D. (1997). *Client teaching guides for home health care* (2nd ed.). Gaithersburg, MD: Aspen.

Miller, M. P., Gillespie, J., Billian, A., & Davel, S. (2001). Prevention of smoking behaviors in middle school students: Student nurse interventions. *Public Health Nurs, 18*(2), 77–81.

Scott, H. K. (2000). Community nursing: Screening for hazardous drinking in a population of well women. *Br J Nurs, 9*(2), 107–114.

Waters, J. A., Fazio, S. L., Hernandez, L., & Segarra, J. (2001). The story of CURA, a Hispanic/Latino drug therapeutic community: Community United for the Rehabilitation of the Addicted, Inc. *J Ethnicity Subst Abuse, 1*(1), 113–134.

Web Sites

Alcoholics Anonymous
http://www.alcoholics-anonymous.org/

American Journal on Addictions
http://www.aaap.org/journals/journalindex.html

American Nurses Association
http://www.nursingworld.org/

International Nurses Society on Addictions
http://www.inrnsa.org/

Journal of Addictions Nursing

http://www.lievertpub.com/jan/default1.asp

Medline Plus
http://www.nlm.nih.gov/medlineplus/substanceabuse.html

Narcotics Anonymous
http://www.na.org/

National Institute on Alcohol Abuse and Alcoholism (NIAAA)
http://www.niaaa.nih.gov/

National Organization on Fetal Alcohol Syndrome
http://www.nofas.org/

National Substance Abuse Web Index: National Clearinghouse for Alcohol and
    Drug Information
http://www.health.org/nsawi

Substance Abuse and Mental Health Services Administration
http://www.samhsa.gov/

16

SPECIAL NEEDS OF INFANTS, CHILDREN, AND ADOLESCENTS

KEY TERMS

adolescent health problems
breastfeeding
immunization status

infant mortality
nutritional status
pediatric health problems

INTRODUCTION

Community health nurses play an important role in addressing the special needs of infants, children, and adolescents. This chapter examines the common health concerns threatening these populations and the nurse's role in health promotion and maintenance.

KEY POINTS

1. Community health has an important role in preventing **infant mortality** and morbidity. Community health nurses can:

   A. assess and counsel pregnant women
   B. refer them to prenatal resources
   C. educate them about health, nutrition, food allergies, immunization, and injury prevention

  D. monitor and refer infants to care when needed

2. Low birth weight children and premature children are more likely to die during their first year.

3. Nutritional status of infants and children is a key aspect of nursing assessment, including:

  A. history about feeding
  B. measuring height and weight
  C. education about **breastfeeding**
  D. introduction of solid foods
  E. nutritional status of the mother

4. Socioeconomic factors such as income, education, culture, and religious practices all impact infant and child nutritional status.

5. Community health nurses have a key role in minimizing the impacts of poverty, such as

  A. linking families with resources (food pantries or Women, Infants, and Children [WIC] program)
  B. educating parents about affordable nutrition
  C. advocating for women and children, who are statistically more likely to fall below the poverty line

6. Immunization status is a key component of infant and child health.

  A. Routine vaccinations for infants and children include:
   i. DPT (diptheria, pertussis, tetanus)
   ii. oral polio
   iii. MMR (measles, mumps, rubella)
   iv. influenza in at-risk populations
   v. hepatitis B

  B. Low immunization rates are caused by:
   i. fear of vaccine side effects
   ii. lack of knowledge about diseases vaccinated against
   iii. lack of access to care

7. In performing these tasks, community health nurses need to be aware of and sensitive to cultural health practices and beliefs related to nutrition, wellness, and the like.

8. Major **pediatric health problems** encountered by community health nurses include:

A. failure to thrive
B. effect of direct and indirect exposure to tobacco smoke
C. unintentional injuries
D. lead poisoning (most often among toddlers and preschool children)
E. poverty and homelessness
F. child abuse and neglect

9. Major **adolescent health problems** encountered by community health nurses include:

A. tobacco use
B. alcohol consumption
C. use of illicit drugs
D. pregnancy
E. sexually transmitted diseases (HIV and others such as chlamydia, gonorrhea, HPV, herpes)
F. violence (including sexual violence, homicide, suicide, assault)
G. inadequate nutrition due to eating disorders, pregnancy, or illness

REVIEW ACTIVITIES

Questions

1. Which of the following would be a way that community health nurses could help prevent infant mortality and morbidity?

a. teach a new mother about breastfeeding and sufficient calorie intake for the mother
b. check weight and blood pressure of a pregnant woman
c. provide a pamphlet to a new mother about childhood immunization schedules
d. all of the above

2. Which children are most likely to die during their first year?

a. babies weighing over 10 pounds at birth
b. males
c. low birth weight or premature babies
d. babies who are breastfed

3. An example of how a community health nurse can assist in minimizing the impact of poverty for mothers and children is:

a. performing weight and measurement checks every two weeks

   b.   making sure that a family does not become dependent on WIC

   c.   teaching a family how to prepare nutritious meals on a limited budget

   d.   none of these measures would help minimize the impact of poverty

4. Which of the following is true about children and immunization?

   a.   Children do not need to be immunized today in the United States because antibiotics are available.

   b.   Parents' fears about vaccine side effects may lead to children not being immunized.

   c.   Lack of access does not impact child immunization rates.

   d.   The community health nurse is not responsible for screening for diseases or immunization status.

5. An example of a commonly encountered pediatric health problem is:

   a.   lead poisoning

   b.   obesity

   c.   tobacco use

   d.   pregnancy

6. A commonly encountered adolescent health problem is:

   a.   failure to thrive

   b.   lead poisoning

   c.   sexually transmitted diseases

   d.   adequate nutrition

Critical-Thinking Questions

1. A client in your clinic has a 2-week-old daughter who weighed 5 pounds at birth. According to your assessment the baby has not gained weight. What education activities would be appropriate for this mother?

2. What are some of the socioeconomic factors that impact how children are fed in your family? How do your family practices differ from those of others you know?

3. Your clients are a young couple and their two children, ages 2 years and 2 months. Both parents smoke. What are some basic educational points that you could provide to these parents?

4. At a school clinic screening you talk with 14-year-old Josie. Her height is 5 feet, 5 inches and she weighs 98 pounds. What adolescent health problem or problems might you be encountering? What are some questions you could ask Josie to learn more?

Discussion Questions

1. What are the resources for mothers in your community who wish to breastfeed?

2. A client in your neighborhood clinic needs to receive public food assistance (WIC, food stamps). How do you get this person in touch with these resources in your community?

3. What infant and child immunizations are offered by your local health department?

References

Adams, C., et al. (2001). Breastfeeding trends at a community breastfeeding center: An evaluative survey. *JOGNN, 30*(4), 392–400.

Barnes-Boyd, D., Norr, K. F., & Nacion, K. W. (2001). Promoting infant health through home visiting by a nurse-managed community worker team. *Public Health Nurse, 18*(4), 225–235.

Bekaert, S. (2001). Preventing unwanted teenage pregnancies. *Nurs Times, 97*(19), 38–39.

Brenner, R. A., et al. (2001). Prevalence and predictors of immunization among inner-city infants: A birth cohort study. *Pediatrics, 108*(3), 661–670.

Canino, I. A., & Spurlock, J. (2000). *Culturally diverse children and adolescents: Assessment, diagnosis, and treatment* (2nd ed.). New York: Guilford.

Cohen, S. M. (2001). Lead poisoning: A summary of treatment and prevention. *Pediatr Nurs, 27*(2), 125–126, 147–148.

Craft-Rosenberg, M., & Denehy, J. (Eds.). (2001). *Nursing interventions for infants, children, and families*. Thousand Oaks, CA: Sage.

Durmont, M. P. (2000). Lead, mental health, and social action: A view from the bridge. *Public Health Rep, 115*(6), 505–510.

Evers, D. B. (2001). Teaching mothers about childhood immunizations. *MCN, 26*(5), 253–256.

Johnson, M. O. (2001). Meeting health care needs of a vulnerable population: Perceived barriers. *J Community Health Nurs, 18*(1), 35–52.

Karp, R., et al. (2001). Should we screen for lead poisoning after 36 months of age? Experience in the inner city. *Ambulatory Pediatr, 1*(5), 256–258.

Kingon, Y. S., & O'Sullivan, A. L. (2001). The family as a protective asset in adolescent development. *J Holistic Nurs, 19*(2), 102–126.

National Center for Health Statistics. Division of Vital Statistics. (Annual). *Vital statistics of the United States*. Washington, DC: U.S. Government Printing Office.

Pillitteri, A. (1999a). *Child health nursing: Care of the child and family*. Philadelphia: Lippincott, Williams & Wilkins.

Pillitteri, A. (1999b). *Maternal and child health nursing: Care of the child and childbearing family* (3rd ed.). Philadelphia: Lippincott, Williams & Wilkins.

Pugh, L. C., Milligan, R. A., & Brown, L. P. (2001). The breastfeeding support team for low-income, predominantly minority women: A pilot intervention study. *Health Care Women Int, 22*(5), 501–515.

Scheuring, S. E., Hanna, S., & D'Aquila-Lloyd, E. (2001). Strengthening the safety net for adolescent health: Partners in creating realities out of opportunities. *Fam Community Health, 23*(2), 43–53.

Slutsky, P., & Bryant-Stephens, T. (2001). Developing a comprehensive, community-based asthma education and training program. *Pediatr Nurs, 27*(5), 455–457, 461.

Thompson, R., & Emslie, A. (2000). Young children and the risk of accidental injury: Running an audit at nine months. *Community Pract, 73*(10), 799–800.

Villarual, A. M. (2001). Eliminating health disparities for racial and ethnic minorities: A nursing agenda for children. *J Soc Pediatr Nurses, 6*(1), 32–34.

Vivier, P. M., et al. (2001). An assessment of selected preventive screening among children aged 12 to 35 months in a hospital-based Medicaid managed care practice. *Ambulatory Child Health, 7*(1), 3–10.

Wright, C. M. (2001). Identification and management of failure to thrive: A community perspective. *Arch Dis Child, 82*(1), 5–9.

Web Sites

American Academy of Pediatrics: Child Health and Safety Information
http://www.aap.org/

Archives of Pediatric and Adolescent Medicine
http://archpedi.ama-assn.org/

Association of SIDS and Infant Mortality Programs
http://www.asip1.org/

Center for Adolescent and Family Studies
http://www.education.indiana.edu/cas/

Centers for Disease Control and Prevention Adolescent and School Health
    Program
http://www.cdc.gov/nccdphp/dash/

Issues in Comprehensive Pediatric Nursing
http://www.tandf.co.uk/journals/tf/01460862.html

Journal of Pediatric Health Care
http://www.mosby.com/pedhc/

Kid's Health
http://www.kidshealth.org/

Maternal and Child Home Health Visiting
http://vnavt.com/guide%20for%20maternal_and_child_health.htm

National Certification Board of Pediatric Nurse Practitioners and Nurses
http://www.pnpcert.org/

NCHS Fastats: Infant Mortality
http://www.cdc.gov/nchs/fastats/infmort.htm

National Institute for Child Health and Human Development (NICHD)
http://www.nichd.nih.gov/

National Organization on Adolescent Pregnancy, Parenting, and Prevention
http://www.noappp.org/

Pediatric Nursing Journal
http://www.ajj.com/services/pblshing/pnj/default.htm

Recommended Childhood Immunization Schedule
http://www.cdc.gov/nip/recs/child-schedule.pdf

Society for Adolescent Medicine (SAM)
http://www.adolescenthealth.org/

United Nations Economic and Social Development Index
http://www.un.org/esa/subindex/pj10.htm

Part IV

Special Concerns of Community Health Nurses

CHAPTER 17

NUTRITION

INTRODUCTION

Basic nutrition for all age groups is a key foundation for health. Each group has different needs for nutrients and caloric intake, and each group has specific nutritional challenges. Nurses provide nutritional assessment for all these populations, and screening to detect possible nutritional deficits and direct interventions. This chapter reviews key concepts in nutrition, and the nurse's role in promoting adequate nutrition.

KEY POINTS

1. Nutritional needs of young and middle adulthood focus on

    A. appropriate caloric and nutritional intake, particularly with busy schedules

    B. nutrition for women during childbearing years

    C. controlling **obesity,** a major factor affecting health status in later years

    D. assessment of use of alcohol, caffeine, tobacco

E.   assessment of dieting or other weight control measures that do not provide proper nutrients

F.   any diet restrictions for medical reasons

2. **Risk factors** can prevent proper nutrition. These include:

A.   overeating

B.   lack of exercise

C.   poor nutrient content of food (many fast or highly processed foods; foods with high sugar or fat content and low vitamin/mineral content)

D.   chronic illness

3. Older adults are at greater risk for **nutritional deficits** due to:

A.   decreased appetite and sense of thirst

   i.   Taste sensitivity can decrease with age.
   ii. Lack of sense of thirst can lead to dehydration.
   iii. Dehydration can also contribute to lack of taste.

B.   inability to chew properly

   i.   poor-fitting dentures or lack of dentures
   ii. sores in the mouth
   iii. gum disease

C.   constipation

D.   vision loss

   i.   makes food preparation difficult
   ii. loss of aesthetic appeal of food

E.   drug and food interactions

   i.   may decrease appetite
   ii. may cause nausea or diarrhea

F.   chronic illness

   i.   often results in poor appetite
   ii. can cause lack of energy to prepare balanced or adequate meals

4. Community health nurses can provide nutritional assessment for all these populations, screening to detect possible nutritional deficits and then begin interventions.

5. Steps in a **nutritional assessment** include:

A.   Gather data: discuss with client what is eaten, when, how prepared.

B. Compile a food diary for past 24 hours
C. Identify food intolerances or allergies.
D. Provide meal planning.

   i. If another person prepares the food, he or she should be included in the interview.
   ii. Cultural and religious influences on diet should always be considered.

E. Be aware of changes in diet that may confuse clients, as in when they move from hospital to home care.
F. Get information about the client's ability to buy appropriate food.
G. Identify available community resources that are acceptable to the client.

6. The main prevention strategies include:

A. educating patients about:

   i. nutritional challenges
   ii. appropriate nutrition
   iii. strategies to achieve appropriate nutrition

B. providing information about and access to services or support

REVIEW ACTIVITIES

Questions

1. Nutritional factors for young to middle adulthood would include:
a. control of obesity
b. avoiding eating problems due to poor-fitting dentures
c. dealing with vision loss that could affect eating
d. avoiding all takeout or prepared food

2. Which of these conditions could cause an older adult to have nutritional problems?
a. ill-fitting dentures or other mouth problems
b. poor appetite due to chronic illness
c. low vision
d. all of the above

3. In performing a nutritional assessment during a home visit, you need to be sure:

a. that people can cook their own food
b. to ignore complaints about food allergies or dislikes since they inter-
    fere with attaining proper nutrition
c. you have clear and complete information about what the client eats,
    how much, and when
d. that all clients get enough red meat to maintain their iron levels

4. How can chronic illness impact feeding and nutrition?
    a. Chronically ill people complain a lot about their food.
    b. Medications for chronic illnesses can cause side effects that interfere
        with eating.
    c. Most chronically ill people have increased appetites, putting them at
        risk for obesity, a major health risk factor.
    d. None of the above

5. Which of the following would be an appropriate strategy for preventing
    nutrition problems in populations?
    a. sending clients to the hospital for intravenous feeding
    b. gathering data to screen people at risk for nutritional deficits
    c. avoiding use of food pantries or meal delivery because it is best for
        clients to cook their own food at home
    d. all of the above

Critical-Thinking Questions

1. A 70-year-old woman who emigrated from India five years ago is being
    assessed for nutritional needs after she is released from the hospital for
    treatment of influenza. What factors are important in assessing this client?

2. What are some questions you could ask to determine the nutritional status
    of your client, who is 25 years old with three young children?

3. What questions could you ask clients to determine what foods they enjoy
    most, and if they have any food allergies or intolerances?

4. What do you see as the greatest nutritional challenges facing middle-age adults? Name three things a community health nurse could do to assist this population.

Discussion Questions

1. What resources are available in your community for families with children who may not be able to provide for all their nutritional needs?

2. How does your community respond to obesity? According to the local media, what options are available to people? Do these resources have the same focus as a community health approach?

3. Your local YWCA has asked you to speak to caregivers on making sure elders have appropriate nutrition. Make a list of six points that you would cover, and three resources available in your community for these caregivers and elders.

References

Booth, K., & Luker, K. A. (Eds.). (1999). *A practical handbook for community health nurses: Working with children and their parents.* Malden, MA: Blackwell Science.

Bryant, S. A., & Neff-Smith, M. (2001). Risk factors and interventions for obesity in African American women. *Multicult Nurs Health, 7*(1), 54–56.

Chen, C. C., Schilling, L. S., & Lyder, C. H. (2001). A concept analysis of malnutrition in the elderly. *J Adv Nurs, 36*(1), 131–142.

Craft-Rosenberg, M., & Denehy, J. (Eds.). (2001). *Nursing interventions for infants, children, and families.* Thousand Oaks, CA: Sage.

Epke, H. I. (2001). Empowerment for adults with chronic mental health problems and obesity. *Nurs Stand, 15*(39), 37–42.

Garrow, J. S., Ralph, A., & James, W. (Eds.). (2000). *Human nutrition and dietetics* (10th ed.). Edinburgh: Churchill Livingstone.

Hendler, S. S., & Rorvik, D. (Eds.). (2001). *PDR for nutritional supplements.* Montvale, NJ: Medical Economics Books.

Humphrey, C. (1998). *Home care nursing handbook* (3rd ed.). Gaithersburg, MD: Aspen.

Jeffrey, S. (2001). The role of the nurse in obesity management. *J Community Nurs,* 15(3), 20, 22, 26.

Kennedy-Malone, L. (Ed.). (2000). *Management guidelines for gerontological nurse practitioners.* Philadelphia: F. A. Davis

Pennington, J., Bowes, A., & Church, H. (1998). *Bowes & Church's food values of portions commonly used.* Philadelphia: Lippincott, Williams & Wilkins.

Rodwell, S. (2000). *Basic nutrition and diet therapy.* Philadelphia: Mosby Year Book.

Ronzio, R. A. (1997). *The encyclopedia of nutrition and good health.* New York: Facts on File.

Townsend, C., & Roth, R. (2000). *Nutrition & diet therapy* (7th ed.). Clifton Park, NY: Delmar Learning.

Zembrzuski, C. (2001). Try this: Best practices in nursing care to older adults: Nutrition and hydration. *Update,* 23(4), 12.

Web Sites

American Dietetic Association
http://www.eatright.org/

American Heart Association (search for diet)
http://www.americanheart.org/

Food and Drug Administration: Reference Daily Intakes (RDI)
http://www.fda/gov/fdac/special/foodlabel/rditabl.html

Food Nutrition and Consumer Services
http://www.fns.usda.gov/

Journal of the American Dietetic Association
http://www.eatright.org/journal/

Meals on Wheels Association of America
http://www.mealsonwheelsassn.org/

18

FAMILY AND COMMUNITY VIOLENCE

KEY TERMS

acquaintance rape
battering
caregiver overload
child abuse
community violence
elder abuse
emotional abuse
hate crimes
Healthy People 2010
homicide
learned helplessness
mandatory reporting

physical abuse
primary prevention
rape
relationship violence
secondary prevention
sex offender
sexual abuse
sexual violence
stressors
tertiary prevention
violence prevention

INTRODUCTION

Community violence is one of the most urgent problems in the United States today. Violence reduces our overall sense of security and safety within a community or family environment. Nurses need to be aware of the signs of violence, the conditions that foster violence, and steps that can be taken to prevent violence.

KEY POINTS

1. Factors that contribute to violence include:

  A. peer influence
  B. unemployment and poverty
  C. media violence
  D. gun ownership
  E. intrapersonal characteristics
  F. biological factors
  G. family influence

2. Children exposed to **community violence** are deprived of a sense of security and safety. They may also be victims themselves.

3. **Hate crimes** disrupt the lives of the targeted victims and the life of the community as well, by creating fear and distrust among different groups in the community.

4. Nursing research is needed to better understand:

  A. interventions needed for these populations
  B. the underlying causes of violence and its long-term effects

5. Violence against women is a community issue also, due to the high emotional and financial costs.

6. There are many forms of **sexual violence,** ranging from behaviors such as voyeurism to sexual assault.

  A. **Rape** is the most underreported crime in the United States.
  B. **Acquaintance rape,** although it occurs more frequently, is less likely to be reported than stranger rape.
  C. Date rape drugs are increasingly a part of the acquaintance rape scenario.
    i. Drugs most commonly used are Rohypnol (flunitrazepam), Klonopin (clonazepam), GHB, and Ketamine.
    ii. Drugs are generally introduced into the drink of the victim.
    iii. The drugs render the victim unable to resist and sometimes cause amnesia.
    iv. For those who suspect they may have been drugged, blood tests to detect the presence of the drugs can be performed at a hospital emergency room.

    D. Negative, blaming attitudes toward victims still exist in the criminal justice system.

    E. Intervention for victims is needed, in both the short term and the long term. Community health nurses can be essential in finding resources for immediate treatment as well as long-term empowerment and coping skills.

    F. Community health nurses may also work with families in which a family member is a **sex offender.**

7. **Relationship violence** is another key component of family and community violence. This violence can be sexual, physical, emotional, or physical (breaking objects, etc.) and can occur in a number of contexts:

    A. domestic violence
    B. spouse, wife, or partner abuse
    C. battered women
    D. child abuse
    E. elder abuse

8. **Battering** in gay and lesbian relationships is also present, but many victims do not seek help due to fear of bias from the assisting agency.

9. Unable to control outcomes, many victims of domestic violence experience **learned helplessness** resulting in decreased motivation to respond or take action.

10. For community health nurses, identifying victims of violence is the first intervention.

    A. Routine screening for violence or abuse should be part of any health history or assessment.
    B. The community health nurse may also provide intervention for the batterer.

11. **Child abuse** includes physical and sexual abuse of a child and/or neglect.

    A. Children may be vulnerable to neglect or abuse in a household with **stressors** such as

        i. poverty
        ii. substance abuse
        iii. unemployment
        iv. social chaos
        v. adult violence

    B. Severe child abuse is most commonly perpetrated by fathers and by boyfriends of the child's mother.

    C. Some communities disagree as to what constitutes child abuse.

        i. Some cultures are more accepting of corporal punishment, for example, as an acceptable method of disciplining children.

      ii. Adults who were severely punished as children may have a higher tolerance for severe punishment for their children.

    D. The community health nurse must be aware of his or her own biases in this regard when doing assessments and interventions.

    E. Injuries characteristic of **physical abuse** include

        i. burns

      ii. bruises

    iii. fractures

    iv. bite marks or hand imprints on the face or body

    F. The nurse should pay particular attention when the history given does not match the injury sustained.

    G. **Sexual abuse** of children may or may not involve force or coercion, and indicators vary based on the child's developmental stage as well as the child's individual characteristics.

    H. Sexual abuse of male children is believed to be even more severely underreported than sexual abuse of female children.

    I. **Emotional abuse** is the least reported form of abuse; it consists of verbal or behavioral actions that diminish another person's self-esteem and sense of worth.

    J. Differentiating between a child who is emotionally abused and a child who is emotionally disturbed may be difficult since the two presentations are very similar.

    K. Adolescents experience disproportionately high levels of abuse. Warning signs can include:

        i. running away or truancy

      ii. sexual promiscuity

    iii. drug and alcohol abuse

    iv. gang involvement

     v. eating disorders

    vi. self-abusive behaviors

12. **Elder abuse** occurs in 2 to 4 percent of the elder population. It can be physical, emotional, or financial, or a combination.

    A. **Caregiver overload** is believed to be the primary cause of elder abuse. Interventions such as respite care and other support to prevent caregiver overload are the best means of preventing elder abuse.

B. Social isolation puts elders at greater risk for abuse.
C. Elders experiencing abuse are usually reluctant to reveal the abuse because of their fear of retaliation from their caregivers or fear of being placed in an institution.

13. **Homicide** rates in the United States are higher than in any other industrialized country.

    A. Adolescents and young adults are the most likely victims or perpetrators of homicide.
    B. Urban youths have the highest rate of firearm-related homicides.

14. **Healthy People 2010** objectives concerning violence in the United States include:

    A. More education about **violence prevention** in junior high and senior high schools, such as

        i.   peer mediation
        ii. problem-solving skills
        iii. anger management skills
        iv. dealing with diversity
        v.   handling peer pressure
        vi. detecting signs of impending violence

    B. Reduce firearm-related deaths.
    C. Reduce homicides.

15. Most states mandate that health care workers report injuries resulting from crime, intentional violence, abuse, and injuries from weapons. All 50 states require that health care workers report suspected child abuse.

16. The concept of **mandatory reporting** of domestic abuse or violence is controversial, due to the high incidence of retaliation against the victim.

17. **Primary prevention** of family and community violence—the goal is to prevent violence before it happens. Possibilities include:

    A. political activism
    B. networking and building trust and alliances within the community
    C. education and counseling for all age groups, male and female, based on current community situations
    D. providing culturally sensitive education and health promotion
    E. developing curricula in schools and community centers
    F. introducing the topic of violence as part of obtaining a complete history for all adults

G. establishing protocols for dealing with victims and perpetrators of violence

18. Secondary prevention:

A. identifying symptoms of abuse and neglect and providing nursing interventions
B. teaching crisis intervention methods and linking families and communities to available resources
C. coordinating interventions with social or legal services if appropriate

19. Tertiary prevention: working with families who are dealing with long-term consequences of violence

20. Community health nurses dealing with these situations need to make sure of their own support systems and resources, to counteract the stress involved. Good self-care is essential to prevent burnout.

REVIEW ACTIVITIES

Questions

1. Which of the following factors do *not* contribute to violence?
   a. nursing research
   b. media violence
   c. unemployment and poverty
   d. gun ownership

2. A crime that targets a person or persons because of their perceived ethnic or racial makeup is called:
   a. acquaintance rape
   b. child abuse
   c. hate crime
   d. mandatory reporting

3. Which of the following is *not* true about relationship violence?
   a. It can be sexual, emotional, or physical in nature.
   b. It rarely affects women or elders.
   c. It often occurs in the home.
   d. It is the same as a hate crime.

4. A 24-year-old woman in your clinic is being treated for bruises on her face and a broken nose, which were inflicted by her live-in boyfriend. You talk with her about filing charges and contacting a domestic violence shelter but she refuses, saying that these measures "never help." This woman is exhibiting which of the following?

   a.   child abuse
   b.   caregiver overload
   c.   learned helplessness
   d.   primary prevention

5. Of the following factors, which could make children in a household more vulnerable to abuse or neglect?

   a.   poverty and unemployment
   b.   the presence of the mother's boyfriend
   c.   substance abuse
   d.   all of the above

6. Bruises on a child's body that are the size and shape of a human hand could be signs of:

   a.   emotional abuse
   b.   stressors
   c.   physical abuse
   d.   homicide

7. Which of the following is true about sexual abuse?

   a.   It always involves force.
   b.   It always involves females abused by males.
   c.   It always occurs within families.
   d.   None of the above.

8. Verbal remarks that make a person feel worthless are called:

   a.   mandatory reporting
   b.   stressors
   c.   emotional abuse
   d.   physical abuse

9. Which of the following is *not* true about elder abuse?

   a.   Elders often fear retaliation if they tell someone about the abuse.
   b.   It occurs in all except 4 percent of elder-caregiver relationships.
   c.   It is caused primarily by caregiver overload.
   d.   It can be prevented by respite care.

10. A school that wants to educate its students about violence prevention could teach them about which of the following?

   a.   how to give in to violent peers

b. ignoring students who are angry and upset until they learn how to manage their anger
c. problem-solving and anger management strategies
d. how to safely use firearms for protection

11. Teaching children about how not to get into a fight at school is an example of:
a. mandatory reporting
b. primary prevention
c. secondary prevention
d. avoiding responsibility for standing up for themselves

12. Community health nurses who work in communities or populations with high rates of violence are at risk for:
a. secondary prevention
b. burnout
c. peer mediation
d. self-care

Critical-Thinking Questions

1. You are taking a history of a 10-year-old girl as part of a school health screening program. What might indicate that the child has experienced:
    • physical abuse
    • sexual abuse
    • emotional abuse

2. There are a number of warning signs that indicate an adolescent is being abused. List the signs that could be observed by a community health nurse.

3. For the adolescent in question 2, which signs would need to be uncovered through client assessment? What are some questions you could ask to obtain this information?

4. Name three cultural or religious characteristics that can influence perceptions of family or relationship violence.

5. What are some of the short-term consequences of violence in families and communities? What are the long-term consequences?

Discussion Questions

1. What is the incidence of violence in your community?
- child abuse
- elder abuse
- battered women
- rape
- homicide

How are these statistics reported and recorded? Do you think that the statistics are reliable? Why or why not?

2. What resources are available in your community for women who are involved in abusive relationships? How would you refer a woman in this situation?

3. What resources are available in your community for caregiver families who need respite to avoid burnout or overload?

4. What resources are available in your community for teaching elementary and high school students ways to prevent violence in their schools?

5. Has your community experienced any hate crimes (against people or property) in the past two years? If so, against which group were the crimes directed? How did your community react to these events?

6. In general, how does the media in your community handle violent events? Is there a difference in the way various types of violence are reported?

References

Altschiller, D. (1999). *Hate crimes: A reference book*. Denver, CO: ABC-CLIO.

Berlinger, J. S. (2001). Domestic violence: How you can make a difference, real ways to help a victim find safety. *Nursing, 31*(8), 58–64.

Campbell, J. C., Woods, A. B., Chouaf, K. L., & Parker, B. (2001). Reproductive health consequences of intimate partner violence: A nursing research review. *Clin Nurs Res, 9*(3), 217–223.

Clark, R. E. (2001). *The encyclopedia of child abuse* (2nd ed.). New York: Facts on File.

Dunn, P. C., Vail-Smith, K., & Knight, S. M. (1999). What date/acquaintance rape victims tell others: A study of college student recipients of disclosure. *J Am Coll Health, 47*(5), 213–219.

Henderson, H. (Ed.). (2000). *Domestic violence and child abuse sourcebook: Basic consumer health information about spousal/partner, child, sibling, parent, and elder abuse*. Detroit, MI: Omnigraphics.

Humphreys, J. C. (2001). Growing up in a violent home: The lived experience of daughters of battered women. *J Fam Nurs, 7*(3), 244–260.

Lindenberg, C. S., Solorzano, R. M., Vilaro, F. M., & Westbrook, L. O. (2001). Challenges and strategies for conducting intervention with culturally diverse populations. *J Transcult Nurs, 12*(2), 132–139.

Paavilainen, E., et al. (2001). Risk factors of child maltreatment within the family: Toward a knowledgeable base of family nursing. *Int J Nurs Stud, 38*(3), 297–303.

Roberts, A. R. (Ed.). (1998). *Battered women and their families: Intervention strategies and treatment programs*. New York: Springer.

Sandell, D. S., & Hudson, L. (2000). *Ending elder abuse: A family guide*. Fort Bragg, CA: QED Press.

Schwartz-Kenney, B. M., McCauley, M., & Epstein, M. (2001). *Child abuse: A global perspective*. Westport, CT: Greenwood Press.

Sperekas, N. (2002). *But he says he loves me: Girls speak out on dating abuse*. Brandon, VT: Safer Society Press.

Thobaben, M. (2001). Beyond physical care: Mistreatment of elders by family members. *Home Care Provider, 6*(4), 112–113.

Veenema, T. G. (2001). Children's exposure to community violence. *J Nurs Sch, 33*(2), 167–173.

Web Sites

Elder Abuse web resources
http://www.elderabuselaw.com/

Family Violence Department, National Council of Juvenile and Family Court Judges
http://www.ncjfcj.org/dept/fvd

Feminist Majority Foundation: Domestic Violence Resources
http://www.feminist.org/911/1_support.html

National Center on Elder Abuse
http://www.elderabusecenter.org/

National Clearinghouse on Child Abuse and Neglect Information
http://www.calib.com/ncccanch

National Coalition Against Domestic Violence
http://www.ncadv.org/

National Data Archive on Child Abuse and Neglect
http://www.ndacan.cornell.edu/

National Elder Abuse Prevention and Treatment Resources
http://www.aoa.gov/abuse/default.htm

Rape Prevention Information and Resources
http://www4.nau.edu/fronske/brochures/rape.html

CHAPTER 19

TERRORISM

KEY TERMS

alpha radiation
anthrax
beta radiation
biological
blister agents
blood agents
botulism
chemical
choking agents
cholera
encephalitis
explosive
first responder
gamma radiation

incendiary
irritating agents
mustard agents
mycotoxins
nerve agents
nuclear
plague
ricin
rickettsia
SEB
smallpox
terrorism
toxins
tularemia

INTRODUCTION

The events of September 11, 2001 demonstrated that all communities are vulnerable to acts of terrorism. Nurses can play a pivotal role in responding to terrorist incidents as either emergency first responders, or in the ongoing response after an attack. This chapter defines terrorism, explores the role of the community health nurse in responding to a terrorist incident, and assesses possible types of attacks.

KEY POINTS

1. **Terrorism** is defined by the Federal Bureau of Investigation (FBI) as "the unlawful use of force against persons or property to intimidate or coerce a government, a civilian population, or any segment thereof, in the furtherance of political or social objectives."

2. The definition of terrorism contains three key elements:

   A. The activities and use of force are illegal.
   B. Actions are meant to intimidate or coerce.
   C. Acts are committed to support a political or social cause.

3. All communities are vulnerable to acts of terrorism.

   A. Most communities contain a high-visibility target.
   B. Many communities have manufacturing and technical facilities.
   C. Other locations that can become targets for terrorism include:

       i.   public buildings or places of public assembly
       ii.   mass transit systems
       iii. places that have economic, cultural, or historical significance
       iv.   telecommunications facilities
       v.   nuclear power plants
       vi.   water supplies, such as reservoirs
       vii. food supplies, such as food processing plants

4. Community health nurses can play a pivotal role in responding to terrorist attacks. They may be part of the emergency **first responder** network, or the ongoing response after an attack.

5. Most experts recognize five categories of terrorist incidents:

   A. **biological:** biological substances that are adapted for use as weapons
   B. **nuclear:** using alpha, beta, or gamma radiation
   C. **incendiary:** any substance that produces fire
   D. **chemical:** naturally occurring or human-made substances adapted for use as weapons
   E. **explosive:** any substance that produces an extremely rapid release of gas and heat

6. Biological incidents

A. Biological agents that can be adapted and used as terrorist weapons include

    i. **anthrax** (sometimes found in sheep, also occurs naturally in the environment)
    ii. **tularemia** (rabbit fever)
    iii. **cholera**
    iv. **encephalitis**
    v. **plague** (can be found in prairie dog colonies)
    vi. **botulism** (found in improperly canned food)
    vii. smallpox

B. Biological agents pose a serious threat because:

    i. They are fairly accessible.
    ii. They have the potential for rapid spread.
    iii. They carry the potential for causing devastating casualties.

C. Biological agents can be used in these ways:

    i. aerosols (spray devices)
    ii. oral (contamination of food or water supplies)
    iii. direct skin contact
    iv. exposure
    v. injection

D. The most common types of biological agents include:

    i. bacteria and rickettsia
    ii. viruses
    iii. toxins

E. Bacteria and rickettsia

    i. Bacteria are single-cell organisms that multiply by cell division and can cause disease in humans, plants, and animals.
    ii. **Rickettsia** live inside individual host cells and are smaller than bacteria.

F. Examples of bacteria include:

    i. anthrax (*Bacillus anthracis*)
    ii. cholera (*Vibrio cholerae*)
    iii. plague (*Yersinia pestis*)
    iv. tularemia (*Francisella tularensis*)

G. An example of rickettsia is Q fever (*Coxiella burnetii*).
H. Viruses that could be used as biological agents include:

    i. **smallpox**
    ii. Venezuelan equine encephalitis

      iii. hemorrhagic fevers such as Ebola virus and Marburg virus

      iv. Lassa fever

  I. **Toxins** are naturally occurring substances produced by plants, animals, or microbes that are toxic or poisonous. They are not human-made and are often chemically complex.

  J. Toxins considered to be potential biological agents are

      i. botulism (found in improperly canned food)

      ii. **SEB** (staphylococcal enterotoxin B)

      iii. **ricin** (derived from the castor bean plant)

      iv. **mycotoxins** (produced by a fungus)

  K. Routes of exposure for biological agents are inhalation and ingestion. Skin absorption and injection are possible but less likely.

7. Nuclear incidents

  A. Two main types of nuclear threat exist:

      i. use or threatened use of a nuclear bomb

      ii. use or threatened use of a conventional explosive device that incorporates nuclear material (often called a radiological dispersal device [RDD], or a "dirty bomb")

  B. The greatest potential for terrorist threat is the use of a nuclear device for extortion.

  C. RDDs could come in the form of a conventional bomb or something mobile, such as a truck bomb.

  D. Three main types of radiation are emitted from radioactive materials: alpha, beta, and gamma radiation.

  E. **Alpha radiation** has these characteristics:

      i. heaviest and most highly charged of all nuclear particles

      ii. cannot travel more than a few inches by air

      iii. can be stopped by the outermost layer of dead skin that covers the body

      iv. can be ingested through eating, drinking, or breathing contaminated materials

  F. **Beta radiation** has these characteristics:

      i. particles are smaller than alpha and travel much faster

      ii. can travel through tissue but usually does not penetrate inner organs

      iii. can result in skin burns if exposure is significant or prolonged

      iv. can be ingested through eating, drinking, or breathing contaminated materials

      v. can enter the body through unprotected open wounds

G. **Gamma radiation** has these characteristics:
  i. is pure energy and thus is very penetrating
  ii. can travel great distances and penetrate most materials
  iii. can attack all human tissues and organs
  iv. exposure has distinctive short-term symptoms:
    a. skin irritation or burns
    b. nausea and vomiting
    c. high fever
    d. hair loss

8. Incendiary incidents

A. An incendiary device is any mechanical, electrical, or chemical device used to start a fire.
B. These elements can be used singly or in combination, and the incendiary device can be simple or elaborate.
C. Each incendiary device has three basic components:
  i. igniter or fuse
  ii. container or body (can be glass, metal, plastic, or paper)
  iii. incendiary material or filler

9. Chemical incidents

A. Chemical agents fall into five classes: nerve agents, blister agents, blood agents, choking agents, and irritating agents.

10. Chemical incidents: **nerve agents**

A. Nerve agents have these characteristics:
  i. disrupt nerve impulse transmissions
  ii. are toxic in very small amounts
  iii. examples include sarin, Soman, tabun, and V agent
  iv. usually disseminated by aerosol
B. Exposure to nerve agents causes the following symptoms:
  i. eyes: pinpoint pupils, dim or blurry vision, pain made worse by sunlight
  ii. skin: excessive sweating
  iii. muscles: fine muscle tremors; involuntary twitching and contractions
  iv. respiratory system: runny nose, nasal congestion, chest congestion, coughing, difficulty breathing
  v. digestive system: excessive salivation, abdominal pain, nausea and vomiting, involuntary defecation and urination

  vi. nervous system: anxiety, giddiness, difficulty thinking, difficulty sleeping

 C. Nerve agents are watery or like light oil in their pure form and have no odor.

 D. Nerve agents will kill insects, animals, and birds as well as humans. Many dead animals at an incident scene may be a warning sign of the presence of nerve agents.

11. Chemical incidents: **blister agents**

 A. Also called vesicants, blister agents cause severe burns to eyes, skin, and respiratory tract tissues.

 B. They are sometimes referred to as **mustard agents** because of the characteristic smell.

 C. Blister agents readily penetrate clothing and are easily absorbed into the skin.

 D. Blister agents are very toxic: a few drops on the skin can cause severe injury; 3 grams absorbed through the skin can be fatal.

 E. Symptoms of blister agents include:

  i. eyes: reddening, congestion, tearing, burning, gritty feeling; swelling and severe pain of eyelids, eyelid spasm

  ii. skin: mild itching within 1 to 12 hours, followed by redness, tenderness, and burning pain, followed by burns and fluid-filled blisters; most pronounced in warm, moist areas of the body such as groin and axillae

  iii. respiratory system: burning sensation in nose and throat, hoarseness, profuse runny nose, severe cough, shortness of breath; symptoms occur within 2 to 12 hours of exposure

  iv. digestive system: abdominal pain, nausea, blood-stained vomiting, bloody diarrhea; symptoms follow within 2 to 3 hours of exposure

 F. Blister agents are heavy, oily liquids dispersed by aerosol or vaporization.

 G. In their pure state blister agents are odorless and colorless, but impurities give them a dark color and characteristic mustard smell; a garlic-like odor may also be present.

12. Chemical incidents: **blood agents**

 A. Blood agents interfere with the blood's ability to transport oxygen and result in asphyxiation.

 B. Common blood agents include hydrogen cyanide and cyanogen chloride.

    C.   All blood agents are toxic at high concentrations and lead to rapid death.

    D.   Symptoms associated with blood agents include:

        i.   respiratory distress
       ii.   vomiting and diarrhea
     iii.   vertigo and headaches

    E.   Under pressure, blood agents are liquids but in pure form are gaseous.

    F.   Blood agents typically smell like bitter almonds or peach blossoms.

13. Chemical incidents: **choking agents**

    A.   Choking agents severely stress respiratory system tissues, leading to pulmonary edema, which ends in asphyxiation.

    B.   Choking agents include the common industrial chemicals chlorine and phosgene.

    C.   Symptoms of exposure to choking agents are:

        i.   severe eye irritation
       ii.   respiratory distress (coughing and choking)

    D.   Phosgene smells like recently cut hay.

14. Chemical incidents: **irritating agents**

    A.   Irritating agents, also known as riot control agents or tear gas, cause respiratory distress and tearing of the eyes.

    B.   Common irritating agents include chloropicrin, MACE, tear gas, capsicum/pepper spray, and dibenzoxazepine.

    C.   These gases are designed to incapacitate; can also cause intense pain on contact with skin. In some cases asphyxiation can occur.

    D.   Symptoms of exposure to irritating agents are:

        i.   eyes and throat: burning or irritation; tearing of the eyes
       ii.   respiratory system: respiratory distress, coughing, choking, difficulty breathing
     iii.   digestive system: nausea and vomiting with exposure to high concentrations
     iv.   can cause skin pain, especially in moist areas

15. Explosive incidents

    A.   The U.S. Department of Transportation (DOT) defines an explosive as:

        i.   any substance or article designed to function by explosion (an extremely rapid release of gas or heat)

      ii. any substance or article that, by chemical reaction, can function in a similar manner even if it was not designed to function by explosion

  B. Approximately 70 percent of all terrorist attacks worldwide involve explosives.

16. Warning signs and indicators: biological incidents

  A. unusual numbers of sick or dying people or animals
  B. dissemination of unscheduled and unusual sprays, especially out-doors or at night
  C. abandoned spray devices with no distinct odor
  D. biological incidents can constitute a community public health emergency.
  E. depending on the biological agent used, onset of symptoms may be as rapid as four to six hours, or take days or weeks.
  F. for agents that have delayed symptoms, additional risk is posed by migration of infected individuals.

17. Warning signs and indicators: nuclear incidents

  A. detonation or obvious accident involving radiological materials
  B. DOT placards and labels
  C. monitoring devices used by fire departments and hazardous materials teams

18. Warning signs and indicators: incendiary incidents

  A. evidence of use of incendiary devices such as gasoline or rags
  B. remains of incendiary devices
  C. odors of accelerants
  D. unusually heavy burning or large fire volume

19. Warning signs and indicators: chemical incidents

  A. symptoms of nerve agent exposure: similar symptoms in a large group of people
  B. clammy skin and pinpoint pupils are the best symptomatic indicators.
  C. mass fatalities without other signs of trauma
  D. other indicators of nerve agent release include:

      i. hazardous materials or lab equipment that does not belong, or abandoned spray devices
      ii. exposed individuals reporting unusual tastes or odors

    iii. explosions that disperse liquids, mists, or gases
    iv. explosions that seemed to destroy only the explosive device or package
    v. unscheduled dissemination of an unusual spray
    vi. numerous dead animals, fish, and birds
    vii. absence of insect life in a warm climate
    viii. mass casualties without obvious trauma and distinct casualty patterns

20. Warning signs and indicators: explosive incidents

  A. large-scale damage to a building
  B. blown-out windows and widely scattered debris
  C. victims exhibiting the effects of the blast, such as shrapnel trauma, shocklike symptoms, damage to eardrums

21. All health care workers should have as their first concern their own self-protection. Health care workers cannot help terror victims if they succumb to exposure to agents used in terrorism incidents.

22. There are six types of harm that a responder can encounter at an incident:

  A. thermal
    i. result of exposure to extreme heat or cold
    ii. heat travels by conduction, convection, radiation, and direct flame contact.

  B. radiological
    i. Responder should be familiar with the characteristics of alpha, beta, and gamma radiation and their abilities to penetrate.
    ii. Personal protective equipment including self-contained breathing apparatus is essential for responding to radiologic incidents.

  C. asphyxiative
    i. Simple asphyxiants are inert gases that displace oxygen needed for breathing and reduce the inspired oxygen level so that it is not useful to the body.
    ii. Chemical asphyxiants interrupt the flow of oxygen in the blood or to the tissues and prevent proper oxygen distribution through the body.
    iii. Examples of chemical asphyxiants include hydrogen cyanide, cyanogen chloride, phosgene, carbon monoxide, aniline, and hydrogen sulfide.

  D. chemical

      i. Toxic chemicals produce harmful effects based on the concentration of materials and length of exposure to them; nerve agents are an example.

     ii. Corrosive chemicals cause visible destruction or irreversible alterations in the skin at the site of contact; sulfuric acid is an example.

  E. etiological

      i. Harm comes from exposure to a living microorganism or its toxin, which may cause disease.

     ii. Most common examples are biological agents.

  F. mechanical

      i. Harm comes from trauma due to contact with mechanical or physical hazard.

     ii. An example is injury from shrapnel or from objects such as nails contained in the explosive device.

23. Self-protection strategies

  A. time: minimal exposure to hazards
  B. distance: maintaining a safe distance from the hazard area
  C. shielding

      i. Maintain significant physical barriers between self and hazard area.

     ii. Cars, buildings, personal protective equipment can all be used for shielding.

24. Role of community health nurses in terrorism incidents

  A. Nurses may be part of:

      i. crisis management: emergency response team at the time of the incident

     ii. consequence management: long-term support of and response to consequences of terror incidents on the community, after the initial crisis has ended

  B. primary prevention: preventing illness before it occurs. In the case of terror threats, this could include:

      i. teaching people in a community to recognize signs and symptoms of agents used in terror incidents

     ii. teaching people how to protect or shield themselves in case of a terror incident

    iii. helping communities develop their own emergency or safety response plans as well as longer-term plans

iv. providing immunizations against certain infectious agents, if appropriate

C. secondary prevention: recognizing early symptoms of illness, before they become disabling. This could include:

  i. knowledge of the effects of various agents used in terror incidents
  ii. early recognition of treatable symptoms of agents used in terror incidents
  iii. being part of a follow-up team to track people exposed to an infectious agent
  iv. performing assessments of populations to determine risks from exposure

D. tertiary prevention: management of illness or injury to lessen as much as possible the long-term disabling effects

  i. helping people cope with the physical and emotional effects of terrorism
  ii. treating the long-term effects caused by agents used in terror incidents
  iii. identifying resources available to populations to help them cope with the fallout of terrorism

E. Nurses can advocate to help emergency responders and management agencies better understand the needs of a particular community.

F. Nurses can act also as liaisons between emergency personnel and people in a community before, during, and after an incident.

REVIEW ACTIVITIES

Questions

1. According to the FBI, the definition of terrorism contains which of the following key elements?
    a. high-visibility target
    b. lack of use of force
    c. acts committed to support a cause
    d. mass transit systems

2. All communities are vulnerable to acts of terrorism because:
    a. they have structures that can be targets for terrorism, such as mass transit or telecommunications facilities

b. they have no means of protecting the community against attacks
c. they harbor groups with political agendas
d. they are working with the FBI

3. Which of the following statements is true?
   a. Community health nurses have no role in dealing with terrorism because it cannot be prevented.
   b. Community health nurses are involved only in long-term responses to an attack.
   c. Community health nurses cannot be part of an emergency response team.
   d. Community health nurses can be part of an emergency response or an ongoing response effort.

4. Biological agents used in an act of terrorism can:
   a. be placed in an aerosol device
   b. can spread rapidly and cause devastating casualties
   c. can sometimes occur naturally in the environment
   d. all of the above

5. Which of the following would be classified as a biological agent?
   a. smallpox
   b. beta radiation
   c. sarin
   d. blister agents

6. Which of the following describes the properties of gamma radiation?
   a. particles that can travel through skin but not into inner organs
   b. particles that cause no short-term symptoms after exposure
   c. heavy, highly charged particles that do not penetrate the skin
   d. very penetrating particles that attack all human tissue and organs

7. Which of the following best describes incendiary devices?
   a. They are always elaborate and thus very hard to make.
   b. They must contain a chemical agent to start the fire.
   c. They contain a fuse, container, and material that can start a fire and burn.
   d. None of the above

8. Chemical agents include which of the following?
   a. nerve, blister, blood, choking, and irritating agents
   b. nerve, burning, toxic, and explosive agents
   c. irritating, radiation, and dispersal agents
   d. radiation, incendiary, and toxins

9. How do blood agents work?

a. They cause burns and fluid-filled blisters on the skin, which leads to massive infection.
b. They cause asphyxiation by interfering the blood's ability to transport oxygen to body tissues.
c. They cause bloody diarrhea and vomiting, which leads to dehydration and shock.
d. They cause severe respiratory distress.

10. MACE and capsicum are examples of
a. biological agents
b. choking agents
c. phosgene agents
d. irritating agents

11. A device that is designed to release gas or heat rapidly is classified as
a. a biological device
b. a nuclear device
c. an explosive device
d. a chemical device

12. An incident scene that contained rags, a strong smell of gasoline, and signs of a very hot, fast fire would be evidence of:
a. a nuclear incident
b. an incendiary incident
c. a chemical incident
d. none of the above

13. The first concern for health care workers responding to terrorist incident is:
a. tracking down the source of the incident
b. saving evidence for investigators
c. self-protection to avoid succumbing to agents
d. determining protocol about short- and long-term responses

14. A nurse or other health care worker responding to an incident at which there is a possible radiologic release should:
a. stay completely out of the area to avoid contamination
b. not be concerned because most terrorist devices use alpha radiation
c. be concerned about asphyxiants
d. be sure to wear a self-contained breathing apparatus

15. An example of thermal harm would be:
a. exposure to heat from fire that follows an explosion
b. difficulty breathing due to inhalation of blood agents
c. skin damage from exposure to corrosive chemical agents
d. exposure to microorganisms that can cause burning in the eyes and mucous membranes

16. Trauma due to being hit by shrapnel or other projectiles from a car bomb would be classified as:
  a. chemical harm
  b. mechanical harm
  c. etiological harm
  d. shielding

17. Which of the following are self-protection strategies that incident responders should follow?
  a. maintaining as safe a distance as possible from the hazard area
  b. limiting time spent in the hazard area
  c. maintaining barriers such as buildings or protective equipment between the responder and the hazard area
  d. all of the above

18. Secondary prevention for a terror incident would include:
  a. immunizing people against smallpox
  b. tracking people who may have been exposed to an infectious agent
  c. avoiding references to terror incidents because they increase people's stress
  d. helping people cope with the long-term emotional effects of a terror attack

Critical-Thinking Questions

1. As a first responder to an incident scene, you notice that a large number of people at the site are coughing and rubbing their eyes. Others are lying on the ground but you do not see any marks or signs of injury on their bodies. Even though it is an urban scene, you notice that the air smells like someone has just mowed a lawn or field. What do these clues tell you about the incident?

2. As a responder to a possible terrorist incident, you see a number of people sitting on the curbside of a busy city street. There are a number of empty canisters lying around, and the fire department determines that they are not an explosion or radiation hazard. The people look frightened but otherwise they are not showing any signs of physical distress such as skin irritation or difficulty breathing. Should you consider this a hoax and tell the people to go home?

3. You are a community nurse for a large city that has a number of buildings and facilities that are considered possible terrorist targets. What primary prevention strategies could you put in place in this population?

4. As a community health nurse you are providing tertiary prevention services for a community that was the target of a car bomb. Three young people were killed and five others injured, some severely. What actions might you be involved in?

Discussion Questions

1. What possible terrorist targets exist in your community?

2. What kind of information does your community (police, fire, health department, hospital) provide about possible terrorist incidents?

3. How does your community prepare to respond to a terrorist incident?

4. What do you think is the greatest risk for your community? Biological? Chemical? Incendiary? Nuclear? Irritant?

5. Has your neighborhood or community experienced an incident such as an explosion, massive fire, chemical release? If so, how did the community respond?

6. How would you protect yourself in the event of a terror attack in your neighborhood or the community in which you work? For a biological incident? Incendiary or explosive incident? Nuclear incident? Chemical incident?

7. What do you think is the greatest potential threat to your community?

References

Fighting fear: Bioterrorism raises issues of prophylaxis. (2001). *Hosp Empl Health,* 20(1), 8–9.

Gallo, R. J., & Campbell, D. (2001). Bioterrorism: Challenges and opportunities for local health departments. *J Public Health Manage Pract,* 6(4), 57–62.

Henry, L. (2001). Continuing education: Inhalational anthrax: Threat, clinical presentation, and treatment. *J Am Acad Nurse Pract,* 13(4), 164–170.

Leggardio, R. J. (2000). The threat of biological terrorism: A public health infection control reality. *Infect Control Hosp Epidemiol,* 21(1), 53–56.

Myers, F. E., III (2001). Bioterrorism: Responding to militant microbes. *Nursing,* 31(9), 1–4.

Neiderman, S., Sarosi, G. A., & Glassroth, J. (2001). *Respiratory infections* (2nd ed.). Philadelphia: Lippincott, Williams & Wilkins.

Peralta, L. W. (2000). Bioterrorism: an overview. *Semin Perioper Nurs,* 9(1), 3–10.

Salvucci, A. (2001). *Biological terrorism: responding to the threat: A personal safety manual.* Public Safety Medical. Carpenteria, CA http://www.publicsafetymedical.com

Stopford, B. M. (2000). Responding to the threat of bioterrorism: Practical resources and references and the importance of preparation. *J Emerg Nurs,* 27(5), 471–475, 521–526.

U.S. Department of Defense. (2001). *21st century bioterrorism and germ weapons: U.S. Army field manual for the treatment of biological warfare agent casualties.* Washington, DC: U.S. Department of Defense.

U.S. Department of Justice, Federal Emergency Management Agency. (1999). *Emergency response to terrorism: Self-study.* FEMA/USFA/NFA-ERT:SS. Washington, DC: Federal Emergency Management Agency.

WEB SITES

American College of Physicians/American Society of Internal Medicine (ACP-ASIM)
http://www.acponline.org/bioterro/

Association for Professionals in Infection Control and Epidemiology (APIC)
http://www.apic.org/bioterror/

Bioterrorism resources for nurses
http://www.resourcenurse.com/RN/RN/refcenter/bioterr_refs

Center for the Study of Bioterrorism and Emerging Infections
http://bioterrorism.slu.edu/

Centers for Disease Control and Prevention: Bioterrorism
http://www.bt.cdc.gov/

Emergency Nursing World: Bioterrorism Links and Resources
http://enw.org/Bioterrorism.htm

Federal Emergency Management Agency
http://www.usfa.fema.gov

International Council of Nurses
http://www.icn.ch/matters_bio.htm

Medical Library Association
http://www.mlanet.org/resources/caring/resources.html

Medscape Resource Center
http://www.medscape.com/Medscape/features/ResourceCenter/BioTerr/
    public/RC-index-BioT

National Guideline Clearinghouse
http://www.guideline.gov/STATIC/bio.asp?view=bio

Nursing World: Bioterrorism and Disaster Response
http://www.nursingworld.org/news/disaster/

ANSWER KEY

CHAPTER 1: COMMUNITY HEALTH NURSING

Questions

1. c
2. b
3. c
4. d
5. d
6. b
7. d
8. b

Critical-Thinking Questions

1. A community health nurse who empowers people in a community finds ways for them to learn and acquire skills so that they can be active participants in their health care decisions. People who are empowered can be their own advocates in the health care system and, ultimately, create better systems, based on their experiences and knowledge.

An example of an empowered community would be one that uses its knowledge and skills about drug addiction and use to develop a clinic or needle exchange system that serves the people most in need.

The limitations of empowerment could include that it takes longer and is more difficult in the short term than just telling people what to do. It is also difficult to empower people who are unable to acquire the needed skills or knowledge.

2. Upstream thinking tries to identify and change the variables that contribute to poor health of a population while downstream thinking is geared to short-term, individual interventions. So for HIV or TB, upstream thinking

would target the risk factors, such as poverty, drug use, or lack of information, trying to prevent the diseases before they happen. Downstream thinking would include interventions like directly observed therapy to assure that clients with TB take their medication as ordered, every day, under the observation of a public health worker.

The advantages of upstream thinking are that it is proactive and can be part of an empowerment strategy. The disadvantages are that it can take a long time to effect change. Downstream thinking is effective for conditions that need immediate intervention, but it is less holistic and more reactive.

CHAPTER 2: POPULATION-FOCUSED CARE

Questions

1. b
2. d
3. a
4. b
5. b
6. d
7. a

Critical-Thinking Questions

1. A population could learn to recognize its own health needs, then develop skills and strategies to help meet these needs. This could lead to greater participation in decision making about their needs. For example, people in a community could recognize, through data gathering and education, that high blood pressure is a significant health care problem. They could learn about how high blood pressure affects health and ways to help control blood pressure, to increase their participation in health promotion. In turn, they could participate in community or city forums, educating legislators of the need for funding of blood pressure screening clinics, to detect high blood pressure before its negative effects occur.

2. Data could be gathered by surveying people staying in homeless shelters, or from records of treatment at shelters, doctors' offices, or hospitals, or from the people who work with the homeless population. This community's needs include the ability to avoid exposure, and shoes and socks that fit, to prevent illness. They also need care for illness that has already occurred. Program evaluation could include following the population over time to see if the number of exposure-related illnesses decreases.

3. Policy development is key to community health. Both are targeted to populations and focus on prevention.

4. An assets assessment takes into account the strengths and abilities of a particular group—what they do have rather than what they do not have, which is the focus of a needs assessment. An assets assessment of a group of recently arrived immigrants could reveal a number of assets, depending on the makeup of the group—for example, monetary assets, strong familial ties and support, resilience, and work skills.

CHAPTER 3: HEALTH PROMOTION

Review Questions

1. c
2. d
3. c
4. d
5. a
6. d
7. c
8. b
9. d
10. d
11. a

Critical-Thinking Questions

1. Community health nurses influence health behavior and assist in health protection for people in communities by teaching people which behaviors do and do not contribute to health and well-being, and by implementing strategies to help people stay healthy, from research to education to policy management. As with most community health functions, preventing illness and promoting health can be challenging because they go against the usual medical model of reacting to illness. The advantage is that community health nursing can have a significant impact on the health and well-being of populations and communities.

2. Answers will vary. The key point is that community health nurses need to know about illness-related stress, be aware that people and cultures vary tremendously in their reactions to stress, and understand that the nurse can have a pivotal role in helping people deal with the stress.

3. Answers will vary. Key points are that different models may be appropriate for different populations, and that most nurses will, based on culture, education, and temperament, have a preference for one or the other.

4. Answers will vary. Nurses should be able to identify major categories and types of complementary therapies (mind/body, body, energy, spiritual, etc.). The nurse should also recognize that he or she may have formed a bias against some forms of complementary therapies. Nurses should also be aware that different cultures often have different preferred therapies, and that different populations and cultures may have more or less interest or trust in alternative therapies.

5. A primary prevention strategy for TB: educating people about TB symptoms and risk factors, such as through an advertising campaign on television.
A secondary prevention strategy for TB: recognizing that a population, such as homeless people, is at-risk for the disease and providing screening for that group.
A tertiary prevention strategy for TB: treating a person who has TB with appropriate antibiotics, educating to teach people the importance of completing the antibiotic regimen.

CHAPTER 4: THE ROLE OF THE NURSE

Review Questions

1. b
2. a
3. b
4. d
5. d
6. c
7. b
8. d
9. b

Critical-Thinking Questions

1. The roles of the community health nurse as researcher and as educator might overlap in that the data gathered are used to develop research-based practice, which in turn can be effectively used to teach people about prevention or health promotion.

2. The roles of community health nurse as consultant and educator are alike in that both are trying to help a population get the most accurate information

available about a particular topic. A key difference in these roles is the amount of involvement of the nurse as well as how the nurse interacts with the population. A consultant might assist a population in decision making whereas an educator generally would not.

3. Community health nursing and home health nursing are alike in that both may focus on the needs of a particular population and may in fact treat the same conditions. Both tend to focus on prevention measures and maintaining health. They are different in that home health nursing may be part of a traditional one-on-one medical system, whereas community health nursing will not have this role.

CHAPTER 5: EPIDEMIOLOGY

Questions

1. b
2. c
3. d
4. c
5. d
6. a
7. b
8. d
9. c

Critical-Thinking Questions

1. The first step that a community health nurse concerned about the increased number of persons reporting symptoms of nausea, vomiting, and diarrhea after eating in a particular restaurant would be to gather as much descriptive information as possible about time, place, and person characteristics related to the reported symptoms. It is not appropriate to carry out any other actions or interventions until reliable data have been gathered.

2. In an analytical epidemiological study, cohorts of people affected by a health problem are people who have the same characteristics as those affected but who do not have the health problem being studied.

CHAPTER 6: COMMUNITY ASSESSMENT

Questions

1. d

2. b
3. c
4. a
5. c
6. d
7. c
8. d

Critical-Thinking Questions

1. A community health nurse attempting to conduct a community assessment for a neighborhood group with a high incidence of teenage pregnancy and STDs needs to understand the group's culture about authority and sexuality. Since the nurse is an authority figure, if the teens come from a culture where "young people should obey elders or people in authority," they might agree to fill out a survey to avoid being impolite. Or if the teens come from a culture that does not discuss sexual topics openly, the teens may be very reluctant to provide any detailed information on the survey.

2. Answers will vary. Key points are that personal space has very clear boundaries, and that the space differs, depending on the relationship between the people. Personal space comfort also varies according to culture and often gender, with different cultures having varying limits about what is acceptable and what is not. The nurse also needs to be aware of the signals people give when someone intrudes on their personal space: backing away, avoiding eye contact, and so forth.

CHAPTER 7: THE HOME VISIT

Questions

1. a
2. d
3. c
4. a
5. b
6. d

Critical-Thinking Questions

1. The three most common interventions in home health care include helping families deal with stress created by health problems; making referrals for community services; and teaching and educating clients, with the focus on strengths rather than weaknesses. Each contributes to the health of the client by

working to minimize the impact of health problems on the client and family, making sure that they are not isolated, and empowering them to be active agents in their health care.

2. The nursing process steps include assessment, interview, observation, nursing diagnosis, and care planning. A key task for each step would be (you may have additional or different elements):

- Assessment: determining the caregiver's knowledge about asthma
- Interviewing: talking with the grandmother and the two children
- Observing: open windows (as noted), look for ash trays with cigarette butts, look for inhaler/spacer on counter or table, observe cleanliness (allergies to cockroach excrement is a common cause of asthma symptoms)
- Making a nursing diagnosis: risk for (or actual) impaired home maintenance management; risk for (or actual) ineffective management of the therapeutic regimen
- Planning care: education about proper monitoring of respiratory status with peak flow meter, proper use of inhaler/spacer, investigation of resources to assure family has access to health care (many others)

Cultural factors that might affect this situation could include perceptions about smoking, or the perception that cold, fresh air is always good for you. Also key would be to assess the grandmother's role in the family, and the amount of authority she has in health care decision making for the children.

3. Showing appreciation for a gesture of hospitality while refusing the actual gift is a situation many community health nurses will encounter. This nurse is correct in telling the family politely that he or she is "not allowed" to eat on the job. The nurse could offer to take a food sample with him or her, which allows the family to give a gift. The nurse explaining that he or she is, for health reasons, unable to drink coffee is also acceptable; the message can be "softened" by a comment such as that the coffee smells very good and would be delicious if the nurse could drink it. Thanking the family for their gesture is always appropriate.

CHAPTER 8: ASSESSING FAMILIES

Questions

1. c
2. d
3. c
4. b

5. d
6. d
7. b
8. d
9. a
10. c

Critical-Thinking Questions

1. A family of this makeup could fit a number of configurations: extended family, family of procreation, adoptive or foster family, or multiadult family. Each of these family configurations could fit this combination of adults and children, who clearly function as a family unit but do not seem to have traditional marriage ties.

2. The key components of family physical environment include housing and surrounding conditions; any safety or environmental hazards; and the services available. Psychological environment consists of family dynamics, the family's strengths and weaknesses, skills, family members' roles, and their ability to cope. The social environment consists of factors such as religion, race, ethnicity, culture, socioeconomic class, and resources available through the community.

Each of these environments can positively or negatively impact how families perceive themselves, their members, and their place in the community. They are also good ways to look at how effectively or ineffectively families function, and the possible environmental factors that can contribute to family health or illness. None of these components functions independently—they are interactive and dynamic.

3. Family scenarios using these methods of coping could be:

- triangulation: a father asking his son to tell his mother that the father is upset about what the mother said yesterday, instead of speaking directly to the mother
- scapegoating: telling a nurse that John, the youngest son, is the one responsible for all the family problems, because he was caught taking candy from the store
- pseudomutuality: maintaining family status at the expense of family function, such as not sending a teenage child for treatment of her depression because it would "look bad" to the community for the family to have a member who is depressed.

4. For the community health nurse, the advantages of using the NANDA system are its clear categories and its recognition by the larger medical community. The disadvantages of the NANDA system is that it can lack the more holistic focus of the Omaha system.

CHAPTER 9: LEGAL ISSUES

Questions

1. c
2. d
3. c
4. d
5. b
6. a
7. d

Critical-Thinking Questions

1. In this case the nurse, although well-intentioned in correcting a charting error, could be subject to disciplinary action for falsifying records. In this case, the obscuring of the incorrect information could be interpreted as the nurse attempting to be deceitful about the content of the record. This is why using appropriate and approved charting and correction techniques, such as drawing a single line through the erroneous number, is crucial.

2. In this case the client has designated a health care proxy, but has not provided a living will or document specifying care should the client become unable to make decisions. Thus the directives of the health care proxy must be followed, even though they are different from the verbal wishes of the client. You may share the statements his mother made before he arrived, but legally, he has the authority to direct her care if she is unable to do so.

CHAPTER 10: COMMUNICABLE DISEASE

Questions

1. d
2. b
3. b
4. d
5. d
6. a
7. d
8. b
9. d
10. c
11. b
12. a
13. c

14. a
15. b
16. a
17. b

Critical-Thinking Questions

1. The agents for the following conditions would be:

- diaper rash: urine trapped next to the skin
- influenza: influenza virus
- diarrhea: could be any number of agents: protozoa, virus, bacteria
- heart disease: could be agents such as high-fat diet or an agent such as a bacteria that causes heart damage
- chicken pox: the varicella virus
- bronchitis: virus or bacteria

The agents that would not be considered infectious would be those associated with diaper rash, or the nonbacterial agent of heart disease (diet). All other agents are considered infectious.

2. Within the past 200 years, pandemics have included smallpox and measles (before vaccinations), and the influenza pandemic of 1918. Currently, we are facing a pandemic of HIV disease and AIDS.

3. After receiving the positive lab results for hepatitis B for the mother, the baby should be tested and treated or vaccinated. The nurse should also be sure to use standard precautions and teach the mother and other family members about standard precautions and how to avoid transmission of infection. Another key step is to test the mother's sex partner or partners, and to treat family members who have been exposed to the virus.

4. The key teaching points for a community health nurse at an elementary school after an outbreak of head lice at a nearby school would include teaching students and faculty what lice are, what they and their eggs look like, and symptoms of infestation. Another key education point would be preventive steps to avoid getting head lice, and teaching people how to treat head lice safely and effectively if they occur. Finally, since there is somewhat of a cultural stigma associated with head lice, the nurse should make sure people know that anyone can get head lice, and that infection does not mean that people are "dirty" or have poor hygiene.

CHAPTER 11: SEXUALLY TRANSMITTED DISEASES (STDS)

Review Questions

1. b
2. d
3. c
4. b
5. c
6. a
7. c
8. a
9. d
10. c

Critical-Thinking Questions

1. The primary prevention would consist of educating the teenage couple about how STDs can be transmitted through various modes of intercourse and the methods that are most effective in preventing spread of STDs. Secondary prevention would consist of screening the couple for STDs that they may already have acquired. Tertiary prevention would consist of treating the effects of STDs that they had contracted.

2. A male patient complaining of painful urination who is sexually active should be screened for HSV-2 and gonorrhea, and possibly chlamydia. His reply "of course" to the question about his sexual activity can give the nurse information on his attitudes about sexual activity. The nurse would need to follow up with specific questions on sexual partners and practices.

3. The most vulnerable populations for the following STDs are:

- AIDS: sexually active, IV drug users, newborns of HIV-positive mothers
- herpes simplex virus 2: sexually active, young people, newborns
- chlamydia: sexually active, newborns
- syphilis: sexually active, newborns, women
- gonorrhea: sexually active, newborns, child abuse victims, those who have sex with a carrier

People who are sexually active, and newborns infected during gestation or birth are the vulnerable populations all these STDs have in common.

CHAPTER 12: CHRONIC ILLNESS

Questions

1. d
2. d
3. b
4. b
5. b
6. d

Critical-Thinking Questions

1. For a client with insulin-dependent diabetes, physical impacts could include the short- and long-term health complications of diabetes such as neuropathy and peripheral vascular disease. The psychological/spiritual impacts could include the stress of having a chronic illness, the social restrictions that could accompany a diabetic lifestyle and dietary needs, and feelings of isolation. Economic impacts could be the need for frequent doctors' appointments, medical supplies, reduced ability to work, or costs of special diets and medications.

2. For a person living with diabetes or other chronic illnesses, the first line of prevention would be educating the client to monitor the condition and to develop or maintain behaviors that improve the condition or at least do not worsen it, such as losing weight and exercising regularly. Secondary prevention could include regular blood glucose monitoring. Tertiary prevention could include effectively managing complications such as neuropathy or peripheral vascular disease so that the client has the best quality of life.

3. The concept of empowerment can be applied to a client with asthma in a number of ways. Most people with asthma have triggers that can bring on an asthma attack or exacerbate a flare-up. Empowering clients could include teaching them about triggers, helping them discern which triggers are worst for them, and providing support or information to help them control their exposure to triggers. Empowerment rests on the concept that the client knows best what his or her triggers are, and is the person who can be most effective in avoiding or managing them.

CHAPTER 13: MENTAL ILLNESS

Review Questions

1. b
2. c

3. d
4. c
5. b
6. b
7. b
8. c

Critical-Thinking Questions

1. Secondary prevention strategies appropriate for this person include identification of the disorder that is causing this behavior and treatment, with the goal of shortening the episode or decreasing its intensity. Treatment could include providing access to medication, counseling, or both.

2. The primary prevention strategy for occupants of a city jail would be, first, the awareness that this population is at risk. In addition, the nurse could provide education about alcohol and drugs, mental disorders, and intervention after arrest, a stressful event.

A nurse could encounter any mental disorder in a jail or prison setting but most would be disorders associated with drug and alcohol use, or those that cause people to act impulsively or violently.

3. This male would be considered at risk for suicide because he is male, and because of his ethnicity as well as a history of relationship/family violence. The loss of the long-term relationship could place this man at risk for depression or anxiety. There is also a significant risk that he might behave violently toward his former girlfriend.

CHAPTER 14: HOMELESSNESS

Review Questions

1. c
2. d
3. a
4. d
5. b
6. d
7. b
8. b
9. c
10. d

Critical-Thinking Questions

1. Low literacy and the inability to speak English fluently could put an immigrant at-risk for homelessness because lacking these skills can make the person unemployable, or able to find employment only in very marginal sectors, both of which can lead to poverty, the key cause of homelessness. In addition, the inability to write or speak English could make it very difficult for this person to negotiate any assistance that might be available.

2. Two economic and social factors that could put a rural family at-risk for homelessness are loss of job or income and the disintegration of family structure (through divorce or death). Cultural factors that could lower this risk would be available community or family support resources, or support provided by a religious community.

3. Mental illness and deinstitutionalization contribute to homelessness when people discharged from mental hospitals wind up in places where there is not a sufficient support system to meet their mental health and other needs.

4. Three primary strategies for people at risk for homelessness includes assessing the risks of their becoming homeless, working to increase support systems as needed, and advocating to institute changes at a system level.

Strategies for people who have become homeless includes ensuring a safe place for them to stay and eat, providing immunizations, and teaching them about health threats such as HIV and TB.

CHAPTER 15: ADDICTION

Questions

1. a
2. b
3. c
4. b
5. d
6. d
7. b
8. c
9. d

Critical-Thinking Questions

1. Mr. Quinn's risk for alcohol abuse would be considered high. For elders, risk for abuse increases after a significant change in life status, such as the death

of a spouse. In addition, the behavior that the son describes could be attributed to alcohol use.

2. To work effectively with this man, the nurse would need to consider the following:

- environmental: the client's connections with the neighborhood or community, and any family or other sources of support
- behavioral: how this client copes with various stresses and events in his life
- physical: his current health status, illnesses or conditions present, and whether he uses any medications
- emotional: his level of resilience, the amount of stress, the type or degree of mental illness

3. For this client, a primary prevention strategy would be establishing trust and safety and educating her about drug use and abuse, and about the effects and risks of having a spouse or partner who is a drug abuser. Secondary prevention could include assessment of the woman's physical, emotional, behavioral, and environmental status and screening for illnesses that can accompany drug use. Tertiary prevention is appropriate if step two reveals any conditions that need treatment.

4. Answers will vary. The key point is that nurses should be aware that their experiences with alcohol and drug use, either their own or that of a friend or loved one, strongly impact how they feel about clients' drug-related behaviors. For example, a person who rather easily "kicked the habit" might expect that clients will be able to do the same.

5. Answers will vary. Key points are that drug screening is increasingly a part of the health care climate, due in part to the high incidence of substance abuse in the health care provider population.

CHAPTER 16: SPECIAL NEEDS OF INFANTS, CHILDREN, AND ADOLESCENTS

Questions

1. d
2. c
3. c
4. b
5. a
6. c

Critical-Thinking Questions

1. Teaching that would be appropriate to this client would be information about breastfeeding or bottlefeeding strategies as well as making sure that the mother is getting enough nutrition if she is breastfeeding.

2. Answers will vary. Key points are that family and culture strongly influence what foods people consider acceptable and unacceptable, as well as beliefs about nutrition, eating habits, weight, and so forth. Students should be able to name eating or food practices that are unique to their family and to other families. They should also be aware of biases about food choices or eating that may influence how they work with clients.

3. For these parents, key education points would be the effects of direct and indirect cigarette smoke on children, both in the short term (increased respiratory problems) and in the long term (higher risk of lung cancer). The parents could also receive information about smoking cessation, and how to avoid exposing the children to smoke even if the parents do not quit smoking.

4. The health problem that this teenager might be encountering is inadequate nutrition due to a physical problem or to an eating disorder. Questions that might help include asking her how she feels and whether she has been sick recently, what she likes to eat, her eating habits, her weight at an earlier time, or her perceptions about her body.

CHAPTER 17: NUTRITION

Questions

1. a
2. d
3. c
4. b
5. b

Critical-Thinking Questions

1. For this client, the nurse should be aware of possible special nutritional needs after an illness, and that the woman may not have eaten well in the hospital because of her illness or because the hospital was unable to provide foods she prefers based on her cultural heritage. Another factor is whether she can prepare food for herself. The nurse also needs to consider her cultural heritage, which may not accept certain foods normally provided by a home meals service; the foods may not be appetizing to her, either.

2. To determine the nutritional status of this client, the nurse would ask primarily about eating habits, for example, assessing how much the client eats, how often, and what kinds of food on a typical day. The nurse could also ask about tobacco or alcohol use, or the use of vitamins or other supplements.

3. Sample questions about food preferences could include:
"What is your favorite food or meal?"
"Would you rather have *x* or *y* to eat?"
"Are there any foods you dislike or won't eat?"
Questions for determining a client's food allergies or intolerences could include:
"Are you allergic to any foods?" (and if the answer is yes, "Which ones?" "What happens when you eat them?")
"Are there any foods that upset your stomach?"
"Have you ever broken out in a rash after eating certain foods?" "Which ones?"

4. Generally the greatest challenge facing middle-age adults is getting a nutritious diet that is relatively low in fat and that does not contribute to obesity. To assist this population the community health nurse could educate people about nutritious meals that are easy to fix, assessing what factors might interfere with a person eating a healthy diet, and screening for obesity or high serum cholesterol.

CHAPTER 18: FAMILY AND COMMUNITY VIOLENCE

Questions

1. a
2. c
3. b
4. c
5. d
6. c
7. d
8. c
9. b
10. c
11. b
12. b

Critical-Thinking Questions

1. For a 20-year-old girl, signs that she has experienced physical abuse might be burns, bruises, or marks, especially if these are unexplained or seem incongruous with the client's explanation. Sexual abuse could be indicated by the presence of an STD, or sexual acting out by the child. Signs will vary with the child's age and emotional and mental development. Emotional abuse could be indicated by low self-esteem, depression, or acting out. A key point is that sexual and emotional abuse can be much more difficult to determine, since there may be no definitive "marks" or signs.

2. Warning signs that indicate an adolescent is being abused could include physical injuries and self-injury, depression, and running away, all of which could be observed by the community health nurse.

3. For the adolescent who may be abused, assessment could reveal depression, extent or type of self-injury, alcohol or drug use. Questions that could be asked include questions about feeling sad or hopeless (depression); about modes or circumstances for self-injury; and about when or where drugs or alcohol are used.

4. Cultural or religious characteristics that can influence perceptions of family or relationship violence include:

- family and gender roles concerning authority and the parents' role in childraising
- the tolerance of physical punishment as an appropriate means of disciplining children
- the history of the parents, who may tolerate severe punishment more if they were severely punished as children.

5. Short-term consequences of violence in families and communities could include physical injury and family changes (for example, for arrest or incarceration). Long-term consequences include ongoing impairment of family and community function, and increased chance that violent behavior will be carried into future generations.

CHAPTER 19: TERRORISM

Questions

1. c
2. a
3. d
4. d
5. a

6. d
7. c
8. a
9. b
10. d
11. c
12. b
13. c
14. d
15. a
16. b
17. d
18. b

Critical-Thinking Questions

1. These are all indicators of a chemical attack. Chemicals usually produce large numbers of casualties because of their dispersal, and the injured or dead will not show signs of trauma. Respiratory distress and eye irritation are classic symptoms of chemical exposure, as is the presence of unusual odors. The grass or hay odor could indicate the presence of the chemical phosgene.

2. No. This may be a biological incident. A crucial clue is the presence of the empty canisters. In addition, many biological agents do not produce symptoms right away—they can appear in a few hours or even take days or weeks to develop. In this case, sending people out into the community could pose significant risk not only to those exposed at the site but also to the rest of the population, particularly if the people have been exposed to a biological agent, such as smallpox, which is highly contagious.

3. Primary prevention strategies that could be implemented include educating populations about the different types of terrorist threats and agents that exist, and teaching them to recognize signs and symptoms of agents used in terror incidents. Education could also include teaching people to protect themselves in case of an incident, to minimize exposure and possible health consequences. A community health nurse could also work with a community to help them devise a short- and long-term response and health protection plans, which could include immunizing people against certain infectious agents, building or area evacuation strategies and places where people can congregate during an evacuation. In addition, nurses may wish to suggest that people set up a plan with an out-of-area friend or relative each family member can call to report their location in case of a large-scale disaster in which local land phone and cellular phone lines may be overloaded, preventing family members from calling one another, as occurred in New York and Washington, D.C., on September 11, 2001.

4. Tertiary prevention focuses on managing illness or injury from an incident, to lessen its long-term disabling effects as much as possible. For this population, tertiary strategies could include:

- providing services or referrals to victims and survivors to help them deal with the physical injuries from the car bomb and the emotional trauma that follows such an attack. When the victims are young people, the emotional reaction is often more pronounced.
- providing ongoing nursing care to those who were injured and attempting to lessen any current disability and prevent any further disability. In the case of a car bomb, injuries could include trauma from shrapnel, burns, or damage to hearing and sight.
- identifying additional resources for those directly affected by the attack (injured), the families and friends of those killed, and the community at large. These resources would be used to support the recovery of the community and help it deal with the fallout caused by the terrorist attack.

INDEX